homemade
DAIRY-FREE
keto
cookbook

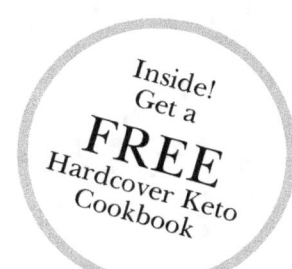

Inside!
Get a
FREE
Hardcover Keto
Cookbook

homemade

DAIRY-FREE

keto

cookbook

Fat Burning & Delicious Meals, Shakes, Chocolate, Ice Cream. Yogurt and Snacks

ELIZABETH JANE

Contents

Lunch (12)

Snacks, Sides, & Sauces (20)

Dinner (19)

Desserts (18)

Drinks (12)

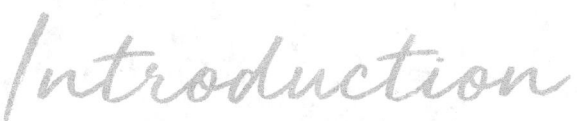

Introduction

Following a dairy-free ketogenic diet can often feel like the fun is taken out of eating. In fact, a dairy-free ketogenic diet doesn't even allow for some of the dairy-delicious treats anymore which is why I was inspired to write this book.

I wanted to create a cookbook that was full of delicious and easy to make keto-friendly desserts that weren't going to knock you out of ketosis. I wanted to create dessert options that you can enjoy without feeling like you are taking a "cheat day."

In this book, you will find 101 mouthwateringly dairy-free keto-approved recipes for every meal, including recipes for breakfast, lunch, dinner, snack, dessert, and even drinks!

I hope this dairy-free ketogenic book becomes a staple in your kitchen and that it brings a little joy back into creating and enjoying some guilt-free dairy substitutions.

Because of your purchase, don't forget to grab your additional, FREE, hardcover ketogenic cookbook that I became famous for at KetoPublishing.com/flavor - Enjoy!

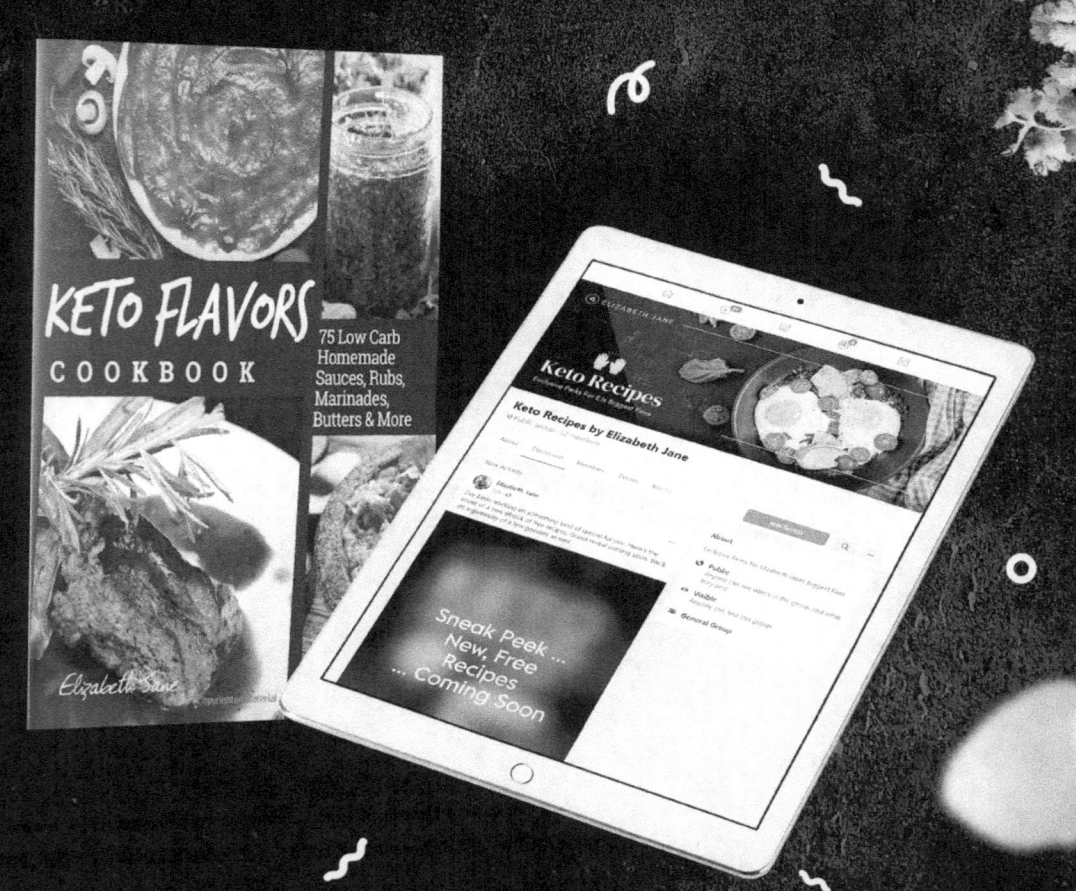
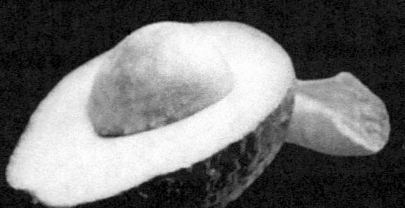

How This Book Works

This cookbook contains helpful cooking tips so that you can make the best dairy-free keto recipes possible! There are also serving suggestions listed to give you an idea about what each of these dishes pairs well with. You will also notice there is a difficulty level and cost scale listed on each recipe. Here is how to read both of these scales to determine the difficulty and price scale for each recipe.

Difficulty Level:

1. An easy-to-make recipe that can be put together with just a handful of ingredients and in a short amount of time.

2. These recipes are a little more difficult and time consuming, but are still easy enough even for beginners.

3. A more advanced recipe for the adventurous cook! You will not see too many level 3 recipes in this book. These recipes are great for when you have a little bit more time to spend in the kitchen and when you want to make something out of the ordinary.

Cost:

$: A-low-budget everyday recipe.

$$: A middle of the road, moderately priced recipe. The majority of the recipes you will find in this book are considered a level $$ on the cost scale.

$$$: A more expensive recipe that is great for serving at a family gathering or party. These recipes tend to contain pricy ingredients. You will not see too many level $$$ recipes in this book, but there are a few that you can make to impress your guests with!

Breakfast

Avocado Veggie Omelet

Prep Time: 10 minutes
Cook Time: 3-5 minutes
Serves: 1
Difficulty Level: 1
Cost: $$

Ingredients:

- 2 eggs
- ½ cup spinach, chopped
- ½ tomato, diced
- 1 tbsp red onion, chopped
- ½ avocado, sliced
- ½ cup arugula
- Coconut or avocado oil for serving

Directions:

1. Start by adding the eggs to a large mixing bowl and whisk well.
2. Add the spinach, tomato, and onion, and whisk again.
3. Heat a medium skillet over medium heat with the coconut or avocado oil.
4. Pour the egg mixture into the skillet and cook for about 3 minutes. Flip half of the omelet over to cover the other side and cook for another 3-5 minutes.
5. Serve with sliced avocado and arugula
6. Enjoy!

· SERVING SUGGESTION ·

SERVE WITH A SPRINKLE OF NUTRITIONAL YEAST FOR ADDED FLAVOR AND PROTEIN.

Nutritional Information:
Carbs: 12g
Fiber: 8g
Net Carbs: 4g
Protein: 14g
Fat: 29g
Calories: 346

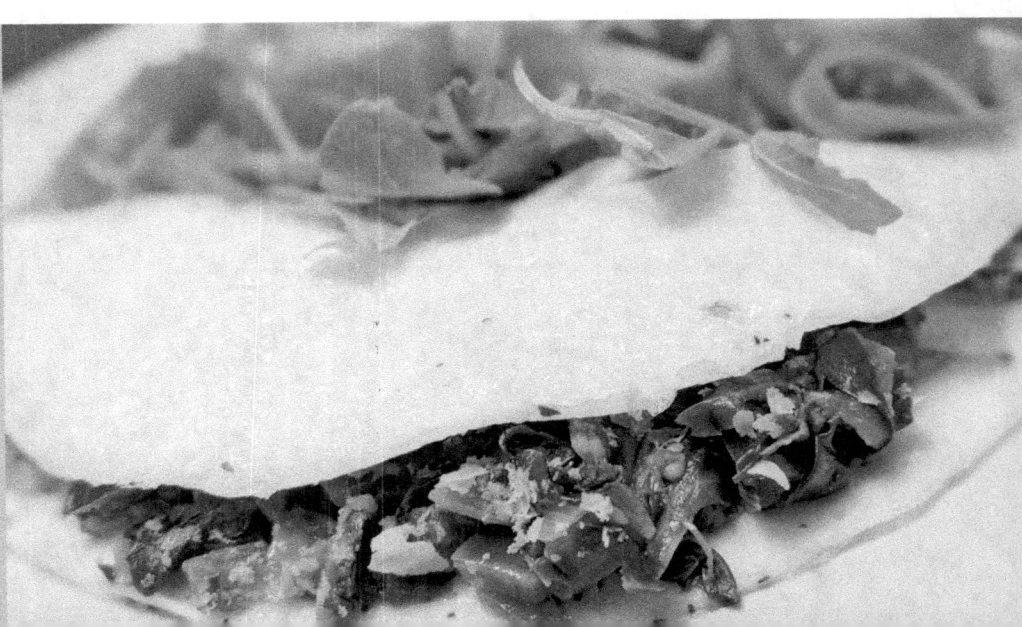

Turkey & Spinach Egg Muffins

Prep Time: 10 minutes
Cook Time: 15-20 minutes
Serves: 6
Difficulty Level: 1
Cost: $

Ingredients:

- 6 eggs
- ½ cup cooked ground turkey
- ½ cup spinach, chopped
- 1 clove of garlic, chopped
- ½ sweet yellow onion, chopped
- ½ tsp sea salt
- ¼ tsp black pepper

Directions:

1. Start by preheating the oven to 350 degrees F and line a muffin tin with 6 muffin liners.
2. Add the eggs to a large mixing bowl and whisk well.
3. Add the remaining ingredients and whisk.
4. Pour the mixture into the muffin tins and bake for 15-20 minutes or until set.
5. Enjoy right away and store leftovers in the fridge.

• SERVING SUGGESTION •

SERVE WITH A SPRINKLE OF NUTRITIONAL YEAST FOR ADDED FLAVOR AND PROTEIN.

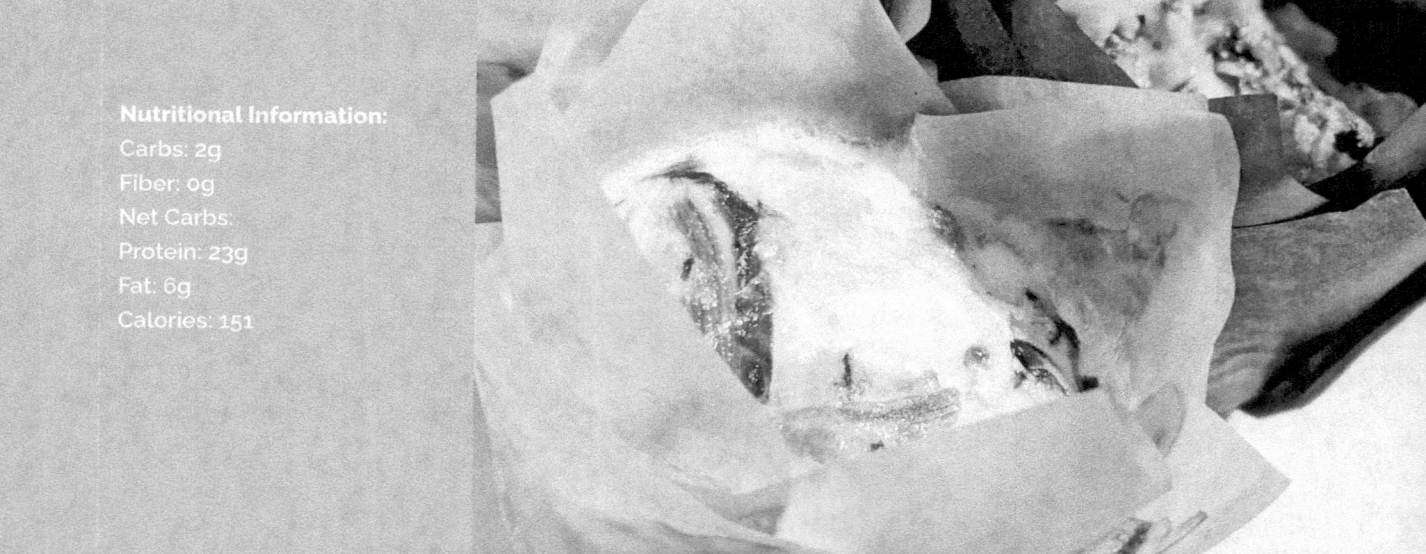

Nutritional Information:
Carbs: 2g
Fiber: 0g
Net Carbs:
Protein: 23g
Fat: 6g
Calories: 151

"Cheesy" Scrambled Eggs

Prep Time: 10 minutes
Cook Time: 5-10 minutes
Serves: 1
Difficulty Level: 1
Cost: $

Ingredients:

- 2 eggs
- 1 splash of unsweetened almond milk
- 2 tbsp nutritional yeast
- 1 tsp garlic powder
- ½ red bell pepper, chopped
- 1 tbsp fresh cilantro, chopped
- 1 pinch of sea salt
- Coconut or avocado oil for cooking

Directions:

1. Start by adding the eggs and almond milk to a mixing bowl and whisk well.

2. Add the remaining ingredients, minus the cooking oil and whisk again.

3. Heat a skillet over medium heat with your cooking oil of choice and add the egg mixture.

4. Scramble and enjoy right away.

· SERVING SUGGESTION ·

SERVE WITH SLICED AVOCADO IF DESIRED.

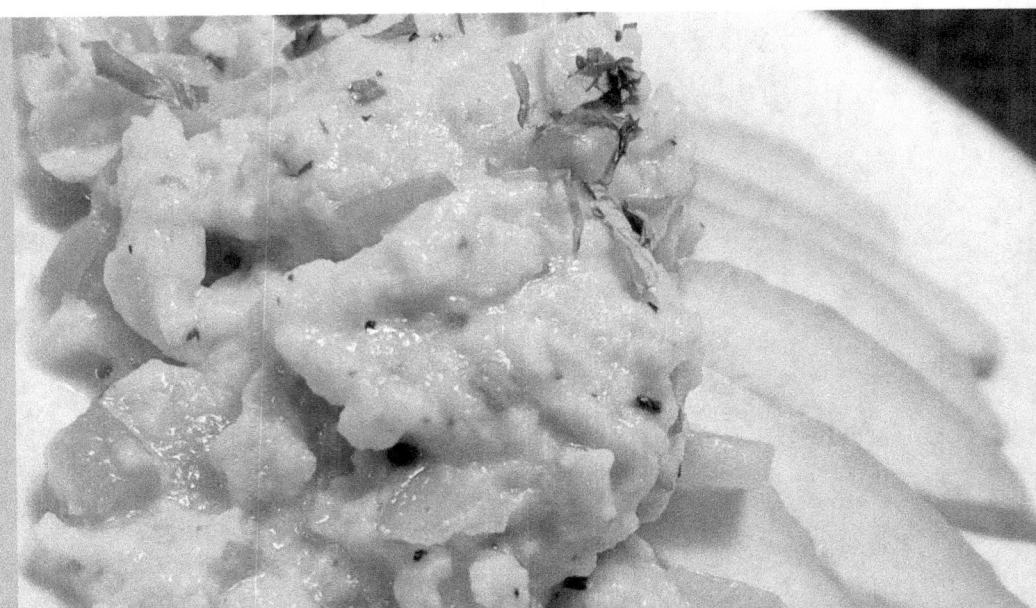

Nutritional Information:
Carbs: 16g
Fiber: 6g
Net Carbs: 10g
Protein: 21g
Fat: 10g
Calories: 225

Stuffed Avocado Halves

Prep Time: 10 minutes
Cook Time: 0 minutes
Serves: 2
Difficulty Level: 1
Cost: $$

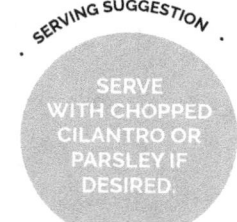

SERVING SUGGESTION

SERVE WITH CHOPPED CILANTRO OR PARSLEY IF DESIRED.

Ingredients:

- 2 eggs, cooked over easy or cooked to your liking
- 1 avocado, halved and pitted
- 2 slices of cooked bacon, crumbled
- 1 red bell pepper, chopped

Directions:

1. Start by cooking the eggs to your liking and add one to each of the avocado halves.

2. Top with cooked bacon and chopped red bell pepper.

3. Enjoy!

Nutritional Information:
Carbs: 14g
Fiber: 8g
Net Carbs: 6g
Protein: 15g
Fat: 32g
Calories: 390

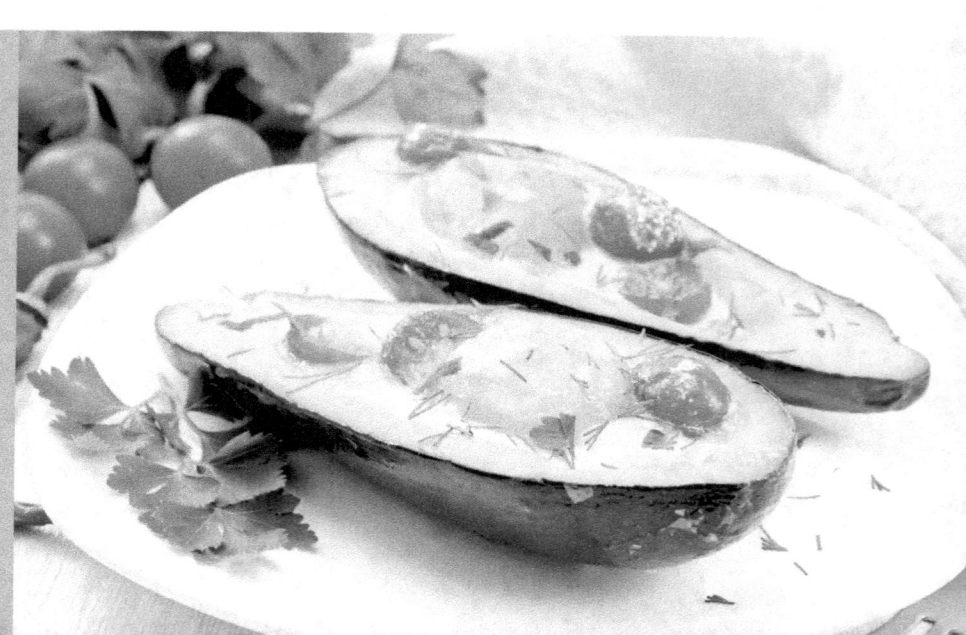

Dairy-Free Raspberry Smoothie

Prep Time: 5 minutes
Cook Time: 0 minutes
Serves: 2
Difficulty Level: 1
Cost: $

Ingredients:

- 1 cup full-fat unsweetened coconut milk
- 1 cup frozen raspberries
- 1 tbsp chia seeds
- 1 scoop of collagen protein powder (optional)

Directions:

1. Add all ingredients to a blender and blend until smooth.
2. Enjoy right away!

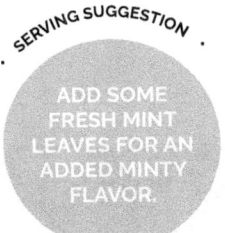

SERVING SUGGESTION

ADD SOME FRESH MINT LEAVES FOR AN ADDED MINTY FLAVOR.

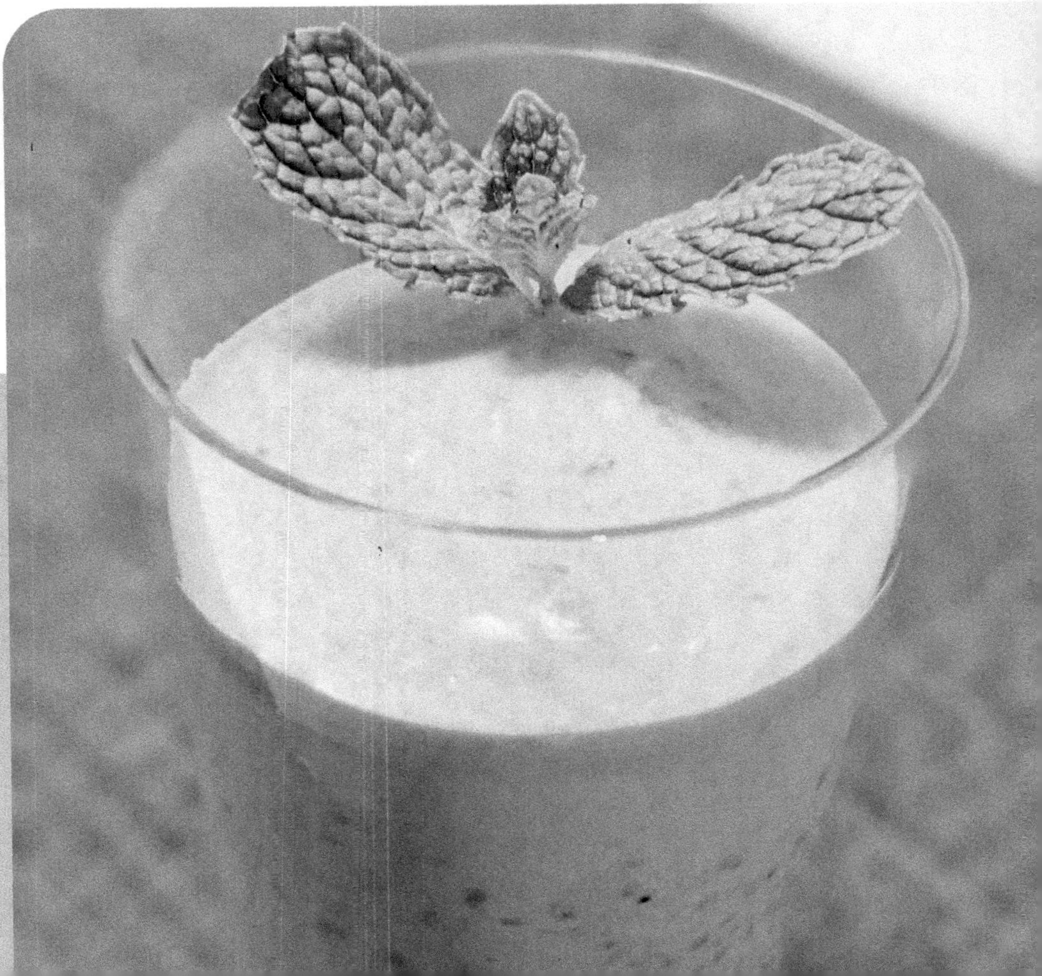

Nutritional Information:
Carbs: 14g
Fiber: 7g
Net Carbs: 7g
Protein: 8g
Fat: 27g
Calories: 304

Orange Coconut Smoothie

Prep Time: 5 minutes

Cook Time: 0 minutes

Serves: 2

Difficulty Level: 1

Cost: $

Ingredients:

- 1 cup full-fat unsweetened coconut milk
- 1 orange, peeled and sliced
- 1 tbsp flaxseeds
- 1 scoop of collagen protein powder (optional)

Directions:

1. Add all ingredients to a blender and blend until smooth.
2. Enjoy right away!

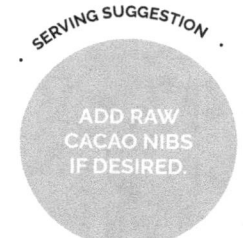

· SERVING SUGGESTION ·

ADD RAW CACAO NIBS IF DESIRED.

Nutritional Information:

Carbs: 19g

Fiber: 6g

Net Carbs: 13g

Protein: 8g

Fat: 30g

Calories: 352

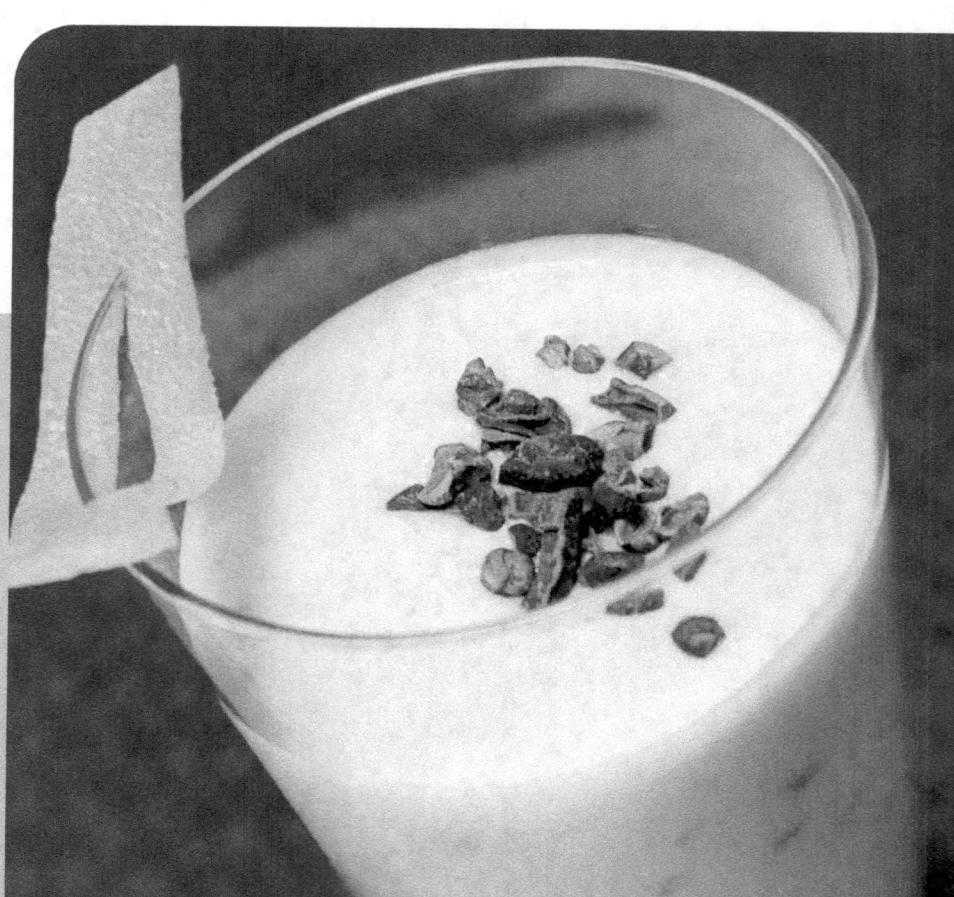

Raspberry Dairy-Free Yogurt Breakfast Bowl

Prep Time: 10 minutes
Cook Time: 0 minutes
Serves: 1
Difficulty Level: 1
Cost: $

Ingredients:

- 1 cup unsweetened coconut milk yogurt
- 1 tbsp chia seeds
- 1 cup raspberries

Directions:

1. Add the coconut milk yogurt to a glass jar and stir in the chia seeds.
2. Top with raspberries.
3. Enjoy!

· SERVING SUGGESTION ·

ENJOY WITH A SPRINKLE OF RAW CACAO NIBS IF DESIRED.

Nutritional Information:
Carbs: 28g
Fiber: 18g
Net Carbs: 10g
Protein: 5g
Fat: 9g
Calories: 194

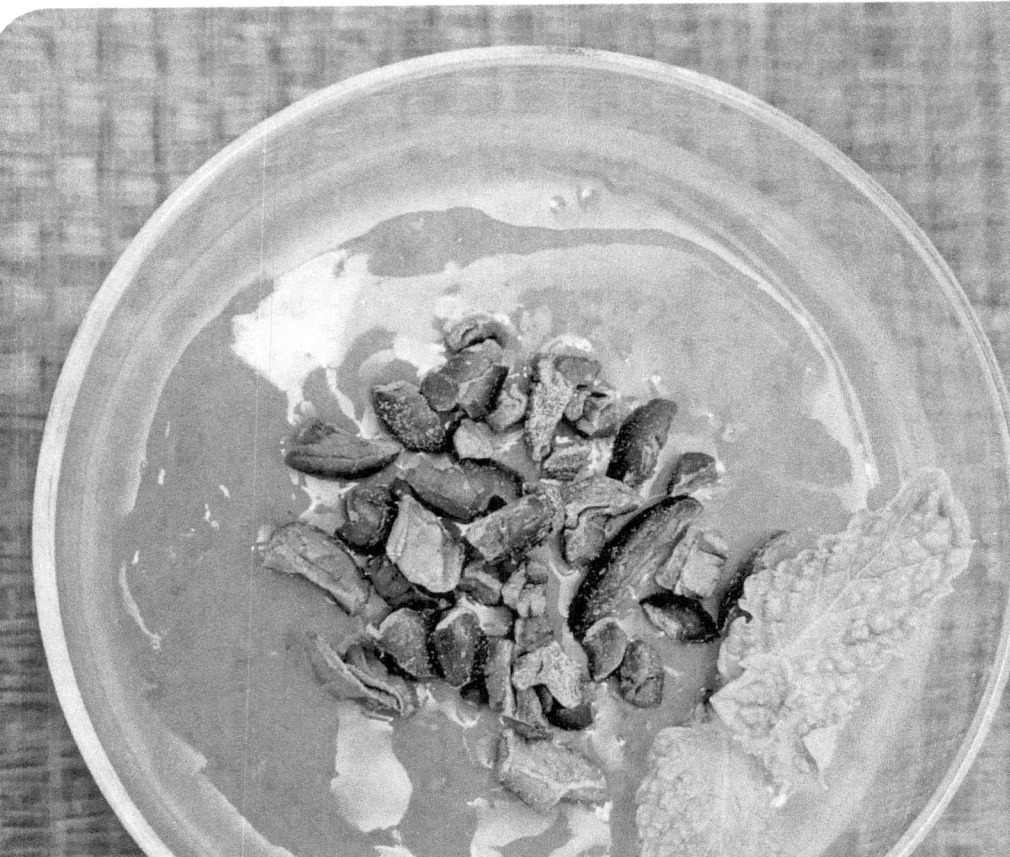

Strawberry Breakfast Smoothie Bowl

Prep Time: 10 minutes
Cook Time: 0 minutes
Serves: 1
Difficulty Level: 1
Cost: $

Ingredients:

- 1 cup frozen strawberries
- ¼ cup full-fat unsweetened coconut milk
- **For topping:** 1 tbsp pumpkin seeds, 1 tbsp chia seeds, 1 tbsp sesame seeds

Directions:

1. Start by adding the strawberries and coconut milk to a blender and blend until creamy.
2. Pour into a serving bowl and top with toppings.
3. Enjoy!

. SERVING SUGGESTION .

TOP WITH FRESH BERRIES IF DESIRED.

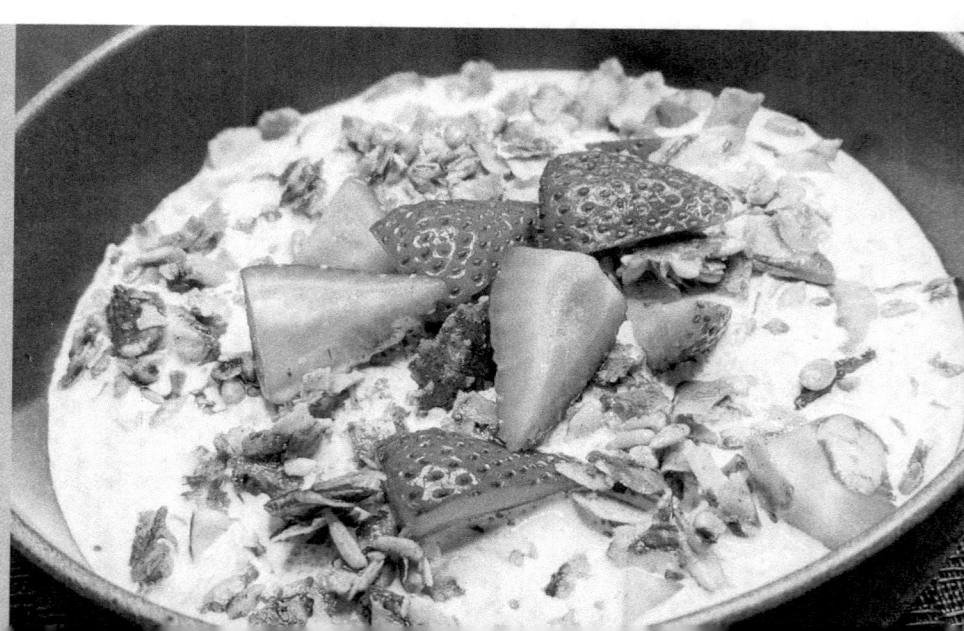

Nutritional Information:
Carbs: 23g
Fiber: 10g
Net Carbs: 13g
Protein: 8g
Fat: 16g
Calories: 239

Dairy-Free Keto Breakfast Coffee

Prep Time: 5 minutes
Cook Time: 5 minutes
Serves: 1
Difficulty Level: 1
Cost: $

Ingredients:

- 1 cup brewed coffee
- ¼ cup full-fat unsweetened coconut milk
- 1 tsp coconut oil
- ½ tsp ground cinnamon
- Zero carb sweetener of choice

Directions:

1. Add the coffee to your favorite mug along with the coconut milk, coconut oil, and cinnamon. Whisk well.

2. Stir in your sweetener of choice.

3. Enjoy!

SERVING SUGGESTION

SPRINKLE WITH EXTRA GROUND CINNAMON BEFORE SERVING.

Nutritional Information:
Carbs: 4g
Fiber: 2g
Net Carbs: 2g
Protein: 2g
Fat: 19g
Calories: 182

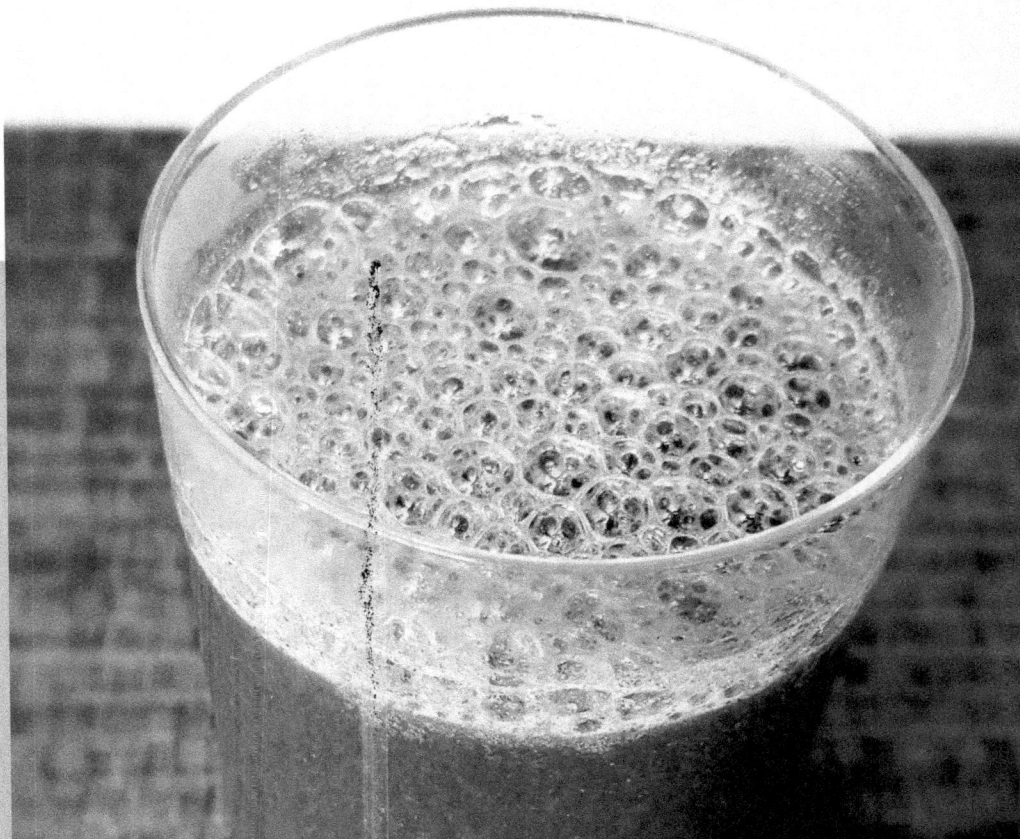

Matcha Breakfast Meal Replacer

Prep Time: 5 minutes
Cook Time: 2-5 minutes
Serves: 1
Difficulty Level: 1
Cost: $

SERVING SUGGESTION

TOP WITH FULL-FAT UNSWEETENED COCONUT WHIPPED CREAM IF DESIRED.

Ingredients:

- ½ cup full-fat unsweetened coconut milk
- ½ cup unsweetened almond milk
- ½ tsp matcha green tea powder
- 1 scoop of collagen peptides
- 1 tsp coconut oil
- 1 tsp pure vanilla extract
- Zero carb sweetener of choice

Directions:

1. Add all ingredients to a stockpot over low heat and whisk until warm.
2. Pour into your favorite mug and enjoy right away.

Nutritional Information:
Carbs: 8g
Fiber: 4g
Net Carbs: 4g
Protein: 13g
Fat: 35g
Calories: 386

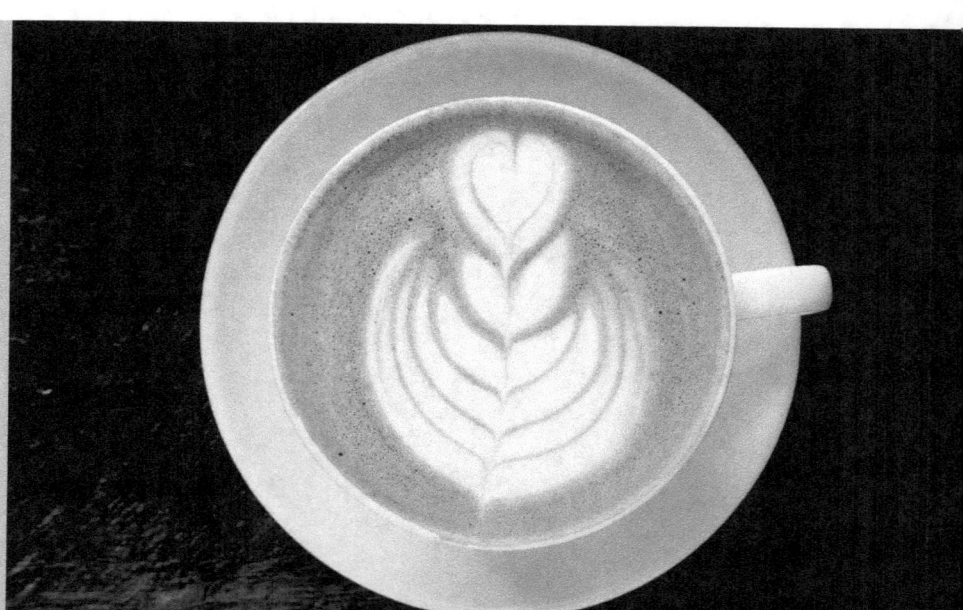

Minty Green Breakfast Smoothie

Prep Time: 5 minutes
Cook Time: 0 minutes
Serves: 1
Difficulty Level: 1
Cost: $$

Ingredients:

- 1 cup unsweetened almond milk
- ½ avocado, pitted and sliced
- 1 handful of spinach
- 1 tsp pure vanilla extract
- ¼ tsp pure peppermint extract
- 1 scoop of collagen peptides

Directions:

1. Add all ingredients to a blender and blend until smooth.
2. Enjoy!

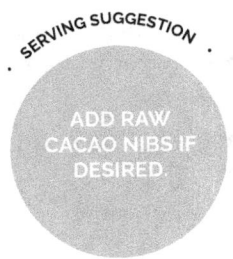

SERVING SUGGESTION

ADD RAW CACAO NIBS IF DESIRED.

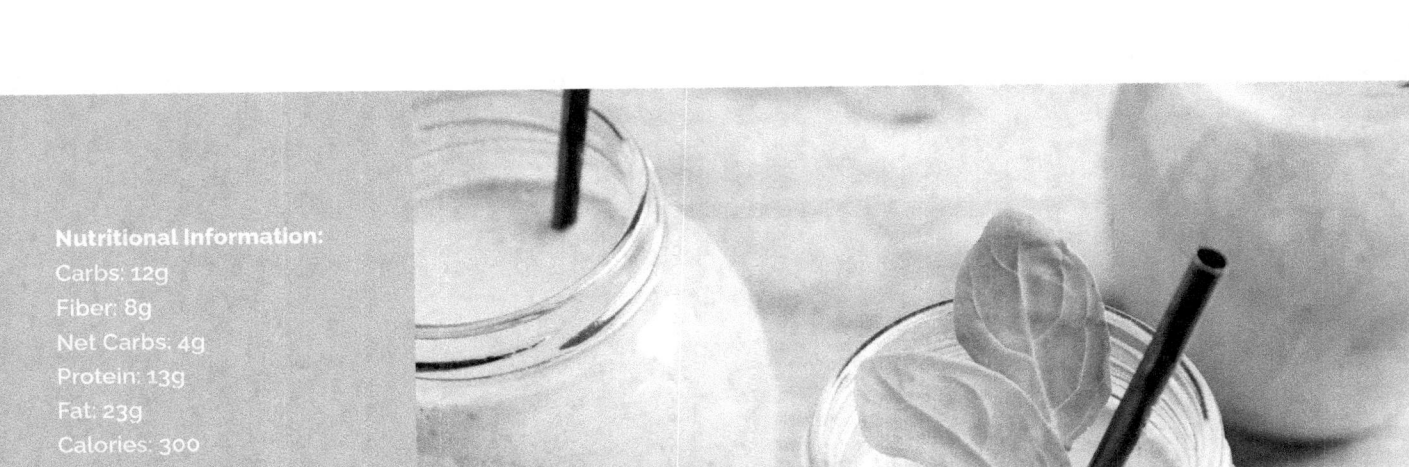

Nutritional Information:
Carbs: 12g
Fiber: 8g
Net Carbs: 4g
Protein: 13g
Fat: 23g
Calories: 300

Bacon & Eggs Avocado Breakfast Sandwich

Prep Time: 15 minutes
Cook Time: 10 minutes
Serves: 2
Difficulty Level: 1
Cost: $$

Ingredients:

- 1 tbsp avocado oil mayo
- 2 slices of lettuce
- 1 slice of tomato
- 1 ripe avocado pitted and halved
- 1 egg, fried
- 2 slices of cooked bacon
- 1 tsp black sesame seeds
- Sea salt to taste

Directions:

1. Start by adding the mayo to one half of the avocado and top with the lettuce, tomato, egg, cooked bacon, and top with the other avocado half.

2. Season with sea salt and sprinkle with black sesame seeds.

· SERVING SUGGESTION ·

SERVE WITH EXTRA COOKED BACON IF DESIRED.

Nutritional Information:
Carbs: 12g
Fiber: 7g
Net Carbs: 5g
Protein: 12g
Fat: 33g
Calories: 380

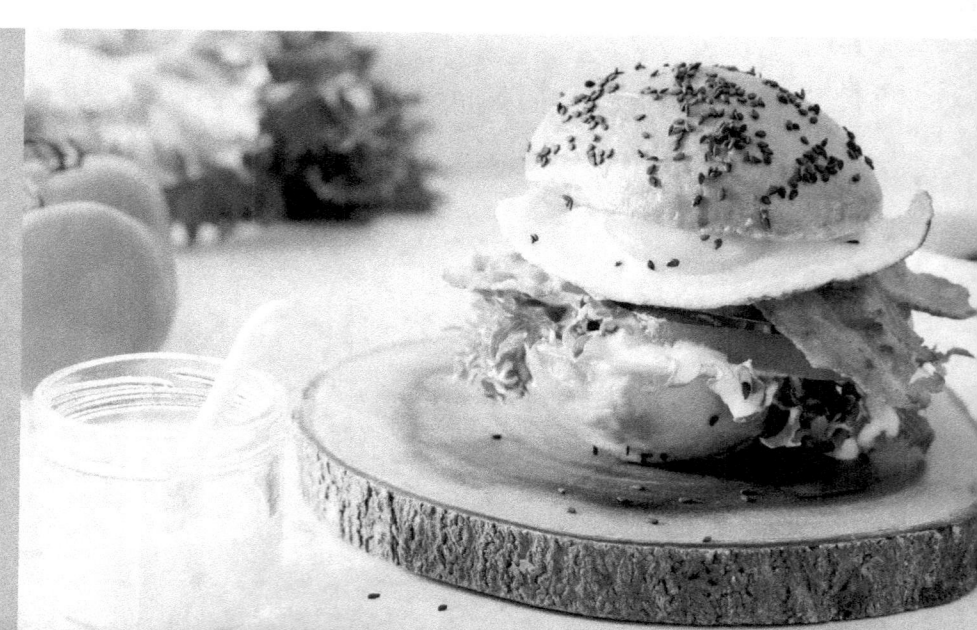

Bacon Wrapped Avocado

Prep Time: 15 minutes
Cook Time: 10-12 minutes
Serves: 4
Difficulty Level: 1
Cost: $$

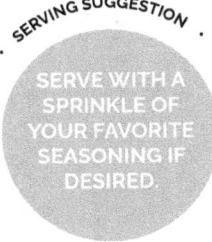

SERVING SUGGESTION

SERVE WITH A SPRINKLE OF YOUR FAVORITE SEASONING IF DESIRED.

Ingredients:

- 2 ripe avocados pitted and sliced into 16 slices
- 8 slices of bacon, cut in half

Directions:

1. Start by preheating the oven to 425 degrees F and line a baking sheet with parchment paper.
2. Wrap each of the avocado slices with bacon and place on the parchment-lined baking sheet.
3. Bake for 10-12 minutes or until the bacon is crispy.
4. Enjoy!

Carbs: 9g
Fiber: 7g
Net Carbs: 2g
Protein: 16g
Fat: 36g
Calories: 411

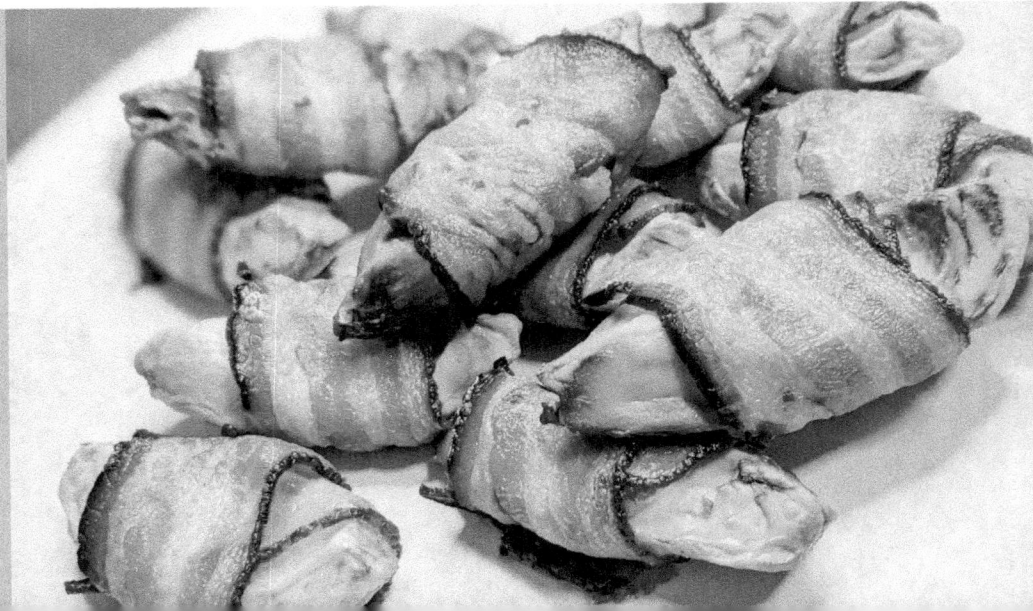

Blender Almond Flour Coconut Pancakes

Prep Time: 10 minutes
Cook Time: 4-8 minutes
Serves: 4
Difficulty Level: 1
Cost: $$

Ingredients:

- 1 cup almond flour
- 1 tsp baking powder
- ¼ cup unsweetened almond milk
- 2 eggs
- 1 tbsp coconut oil, melted
- 1 tsp pure vanilla extract
- 1 tbsp shredded unsweetened coconut
- Extra coconut oil for cooking

Directions:

1. Add all ingredients to a blender minus the shredded coconut and blend until smooth.

2. Add the extra coconut oil to a skillet over low to medium heat and pour about ¼ cup of the batter onto the pan. Cook for about 2-4 minutes on each side.

3. Enjoy with a sprinkle of shredded coconut.

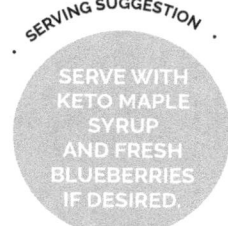

· SERVING SUGGESTION ·

SERVE WITH KETO MAPLE SYRUP AND FRESH BLUEBERRIES IF DESIRED.

Nutritional Information:

Carbs: 3g

Fiber: 1g

Net Carbs: 2g

Protein: 4g

Fat: 10g

Calories: 112

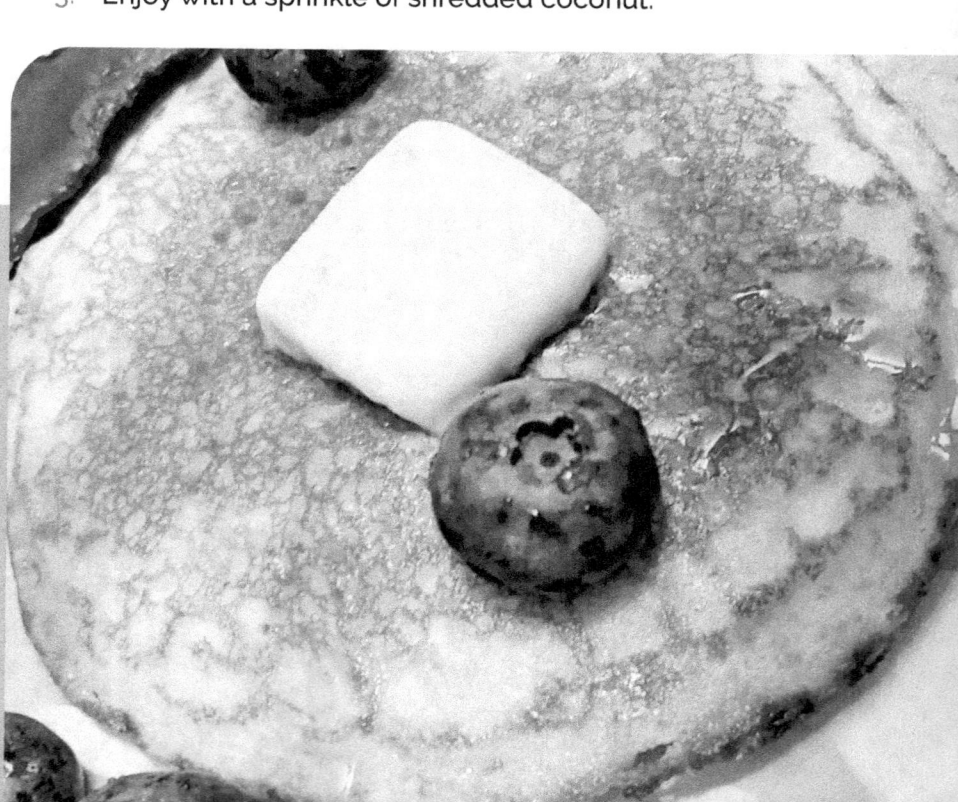

Vanilla Cinnamon Pancakes

Prep Time: 10 minutes
Cook Time: 4-8 minutes
Serves: 4
Difficulty Level: 1
Cost: $$

Ingredients:

- 1 cup almond flour
- 1 tsp baking powder
- ¼ cup unsweetened almond milk
- 2 eggs
- 1 tbsp coconut oil, melted
- 2 tsp pure vanilla extract
- 1 tsp ground cinnamon
- Extra coconut oil for cooking

Directions:

1. Add all ingredients to a blender and blend until smooth.

2. Add the extra coconut oil to a skillet over low to medium heat and pour about ¼ cup of the batter onto the pan. Cook for about 2-4 minutes on each side.

3. Enjoy!

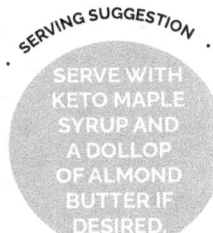

SERVING SUGGESTION

SERVE WITH KETO MAPLE SYRUP AND A DOLLOP OF ALMOND BUTTER IF DESIRED.

Nutritional Information:
Carbs: 3g
Fiber: 1g
Net Carbs: 2g
Protein: 4g
Fat: 9g
Calories: 112

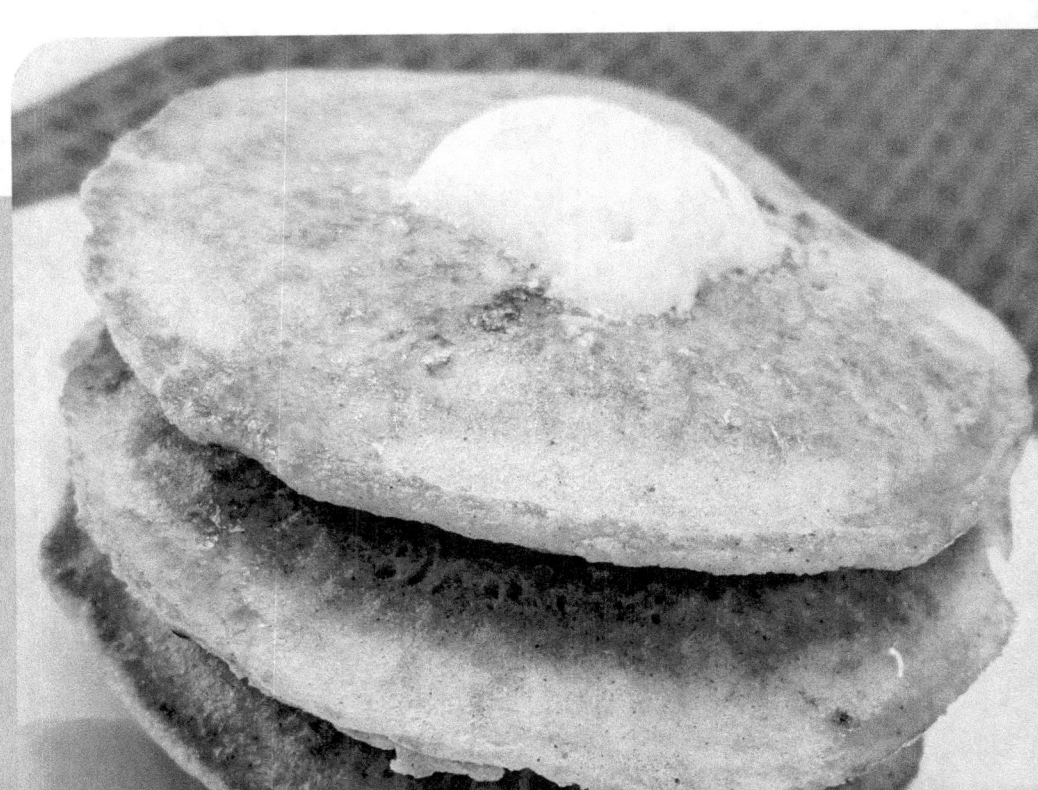

Chocolate Raspberry Breakfast Pudding

Prep Time: 10 minutes + chilling time
Cook Time: 0 minutes
Serves: 3
Difficulty Level: 1
Cost: $$

Ingredients:

- 1 cup unsweetened almond milk
- ¼ cup chia seeds
- 2 tbsp unsweetened cacao powder
- 1 tsp pure vanilla extract
- 1 tbsp erythritol
- ½ cup fresh raspberries

• SERVING SUGGESTION •

SERVE WITH SHREDDED UNSWEETENED COCONUT IF DESIRED.

Directions:

1. Start by adding the almond milk, chia seeds, cacao powder, vanilla, and erythritol to a blender and blend until smooth.

2. Transfer to glass mason-style jars and set in the fridge overnight.

3. Before enjoying, top with fresh raspberries.

4. Enjoy!

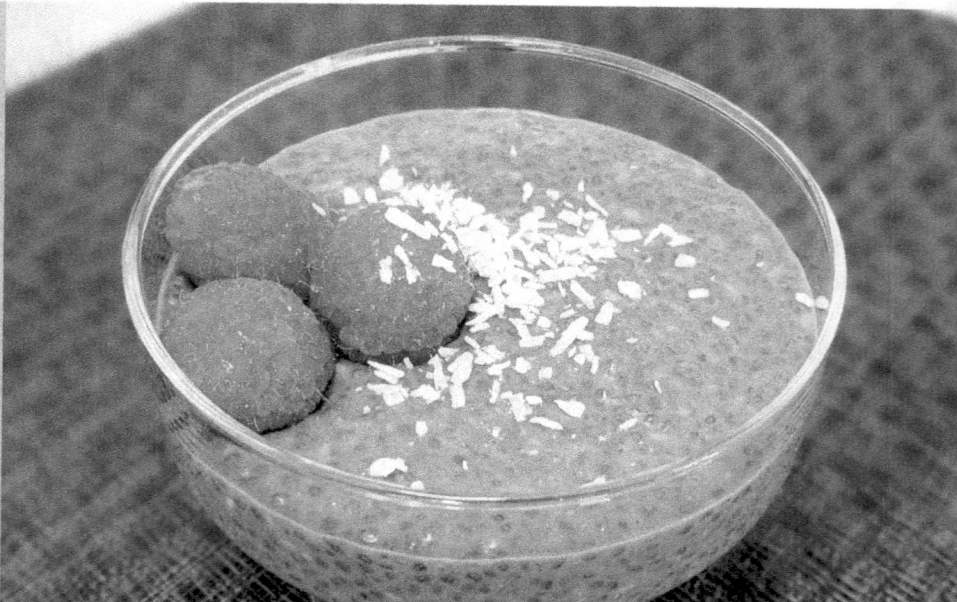

Nutritional Information:

Carbs: 24g

Fiber: 14g

Net Carbs: 10g

Protein: 7g

Fat: 10g

Calories: 155

Superfood Blueberry Breakfast Shake

Prep Time: 5 minutes
Cook Time: 0 minutes
Serves: 2
Difficulty Level: 1
Cost: $$

Ingredients:

- 1 cup unsweetened almond milk
- ½ cup frozen blueberries
- 1 cup spinach
- 1 cup kale
- 1 tbsp chia seeds
- 1 tbsp coconut butter
- 1 tsp pure vanilla extract

Directions:

1. Add all ingredients to a blender and blend until smooth.
2. Enjoy right away!

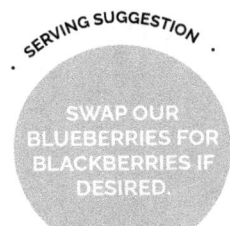

SERVING SUGGESTION

SWAP OUR BLUEBERRIES FOR BLACKBERRIES IF DESIRED.

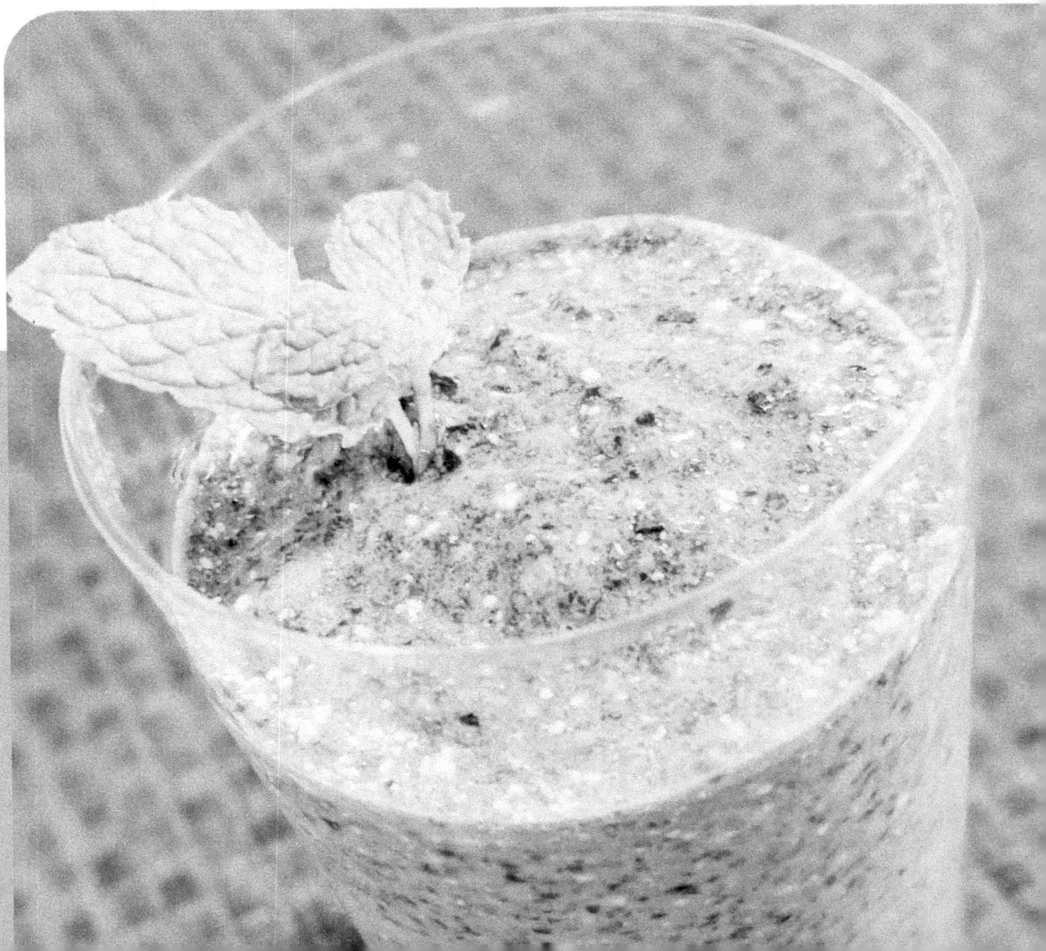

Nutritional Information:
Carbs: 18g
Fiber: 8g
Net Carbs: 10g
Protein: 5g
Fat: 13g
Calories: 195

Vanilla Coconut Protein Yogurt

Prep Time: 5 minutes
Cook Time: 0 minutes
Serves: 1
Difficulty Level: 1
Cost: $$

Ingredients:

- 1 cup unsweetened coconut milk yogurt
- 5 drops of liquid vanilla stevia (or 1 serving according to package directions)
- 1 scoop of collagen peptides
- 1 tsp pure vanilla extract

Directions:

1. Add all ingredients to a mixing bowl and stir well to combine.
2. Enjoy right away!

· SERVING SUGGESTION ·

TOP WITH BLUEBERRIES, RAW CACAO NIBS, AND SHREDDED UNSWEETENED COCONUT IF DESIRED.

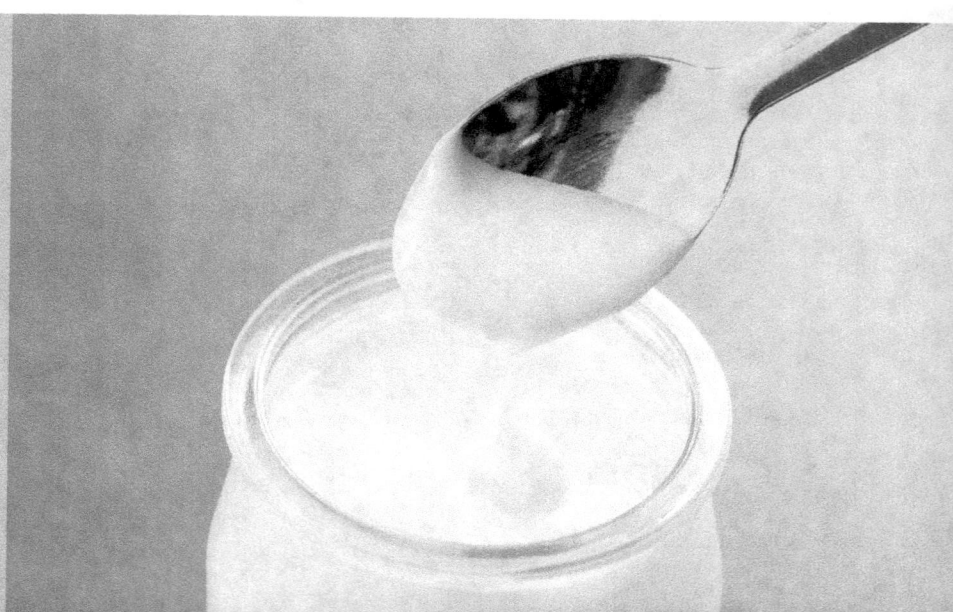

Nutritional Information:
Carbs: 7g
Fiber: 4g
Net Carbs: 3g
Protein: 9g
Fat: 4g
Calories: 98

Chocolate Breakfast Fat Bombs

Prep Time: 15 minutes
+ chilling time
Cook Time: 0 minutes
Serves: 10 (1 fat bomb
per serving)
Difficulty Level: 1
Cost: $$

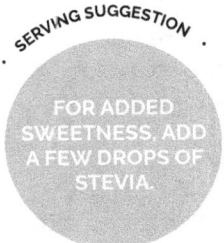

· SERVING SUGGESTION ·

FOR ADDED
SWEETNESS, ADD
A FEW DROPS OF
STEVIA.

Ingredients:

- 1 cup raw cashews
- 1 tbsp shredded unsweetened coconut
- ¼ cup unsweetened cacao powder
- 1 cup almond butter
- 1 tsp pure vanilla extract
- ½ tsp sea salt
- Water as needed

Directions:

1. Start by adding the cashews, shredded coconut, and cacao powder to a high-speed blender or food processor and pulse for 20 seconds.

2. Add the remaining ingredients along with two tablespoons of water to start. Blend until the mixture comes together, adding more water as needed.

3. Transfer to a bowl and set in the fridge for 20 minutes before rolling into bite-sized rounds.

4. Store in the fridge until ready to enjoy.

Nutritional Information:
Carbs: 14g
Fiber: 4g
Net Carbs: 10g
Protein: 8g
Fat: 23g
Calories: 260

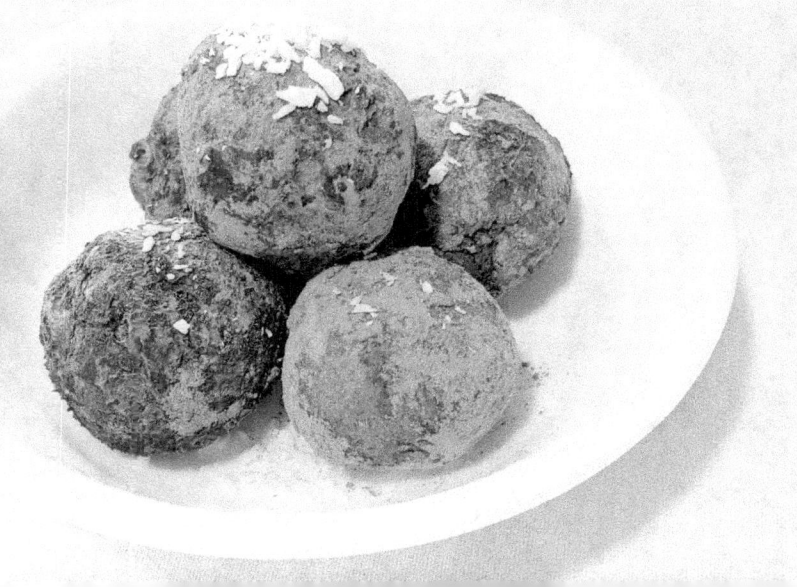

Decadent Chocolate Coconut Breakfast Energy Bites

Prep Time: 15 minutes + chilling time
Cook Time: 0 minutes
Serves: 12 (1 fat bomb per serving)
Difficulty Level: 1
Cost: $$

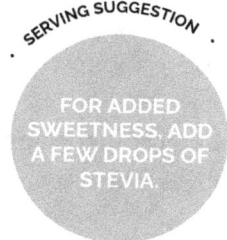

SERVING SUGGESTION

FOR ADDED SWEETNESS, ADD A FEW DROPS OF STEVIA.

Ingredients:

- 1 cup raw cashews
- 1 cup coconut butter
- ¼ cup unsweetened cacao powder + extra for dusting
- 1 tsp pure vanilla extract
- ½ tsp sea salt
- Water as needed

Directions:

1. Start by adding the cashews and cacao powder to a high-speed blender or food processor and pulse for 20 seconds.

2. Add the remaining ingredients (minus the extra cacao powder) along with two tablespoons of water to start. Blend until the mixture comes together, adding more water as needed.

3. Transfer to a bowl and set in the fridge for 20 minutes before rolling into bite-sized rounds and roll into the extra cacao powder.

4. Store in the fridge until ready to enjoy.

Nutritional Information:
Carbs: 16g
Fiber: 9g
Net Carbs: 7g
Protein: 6g
Fat: 31g
Calories: 331

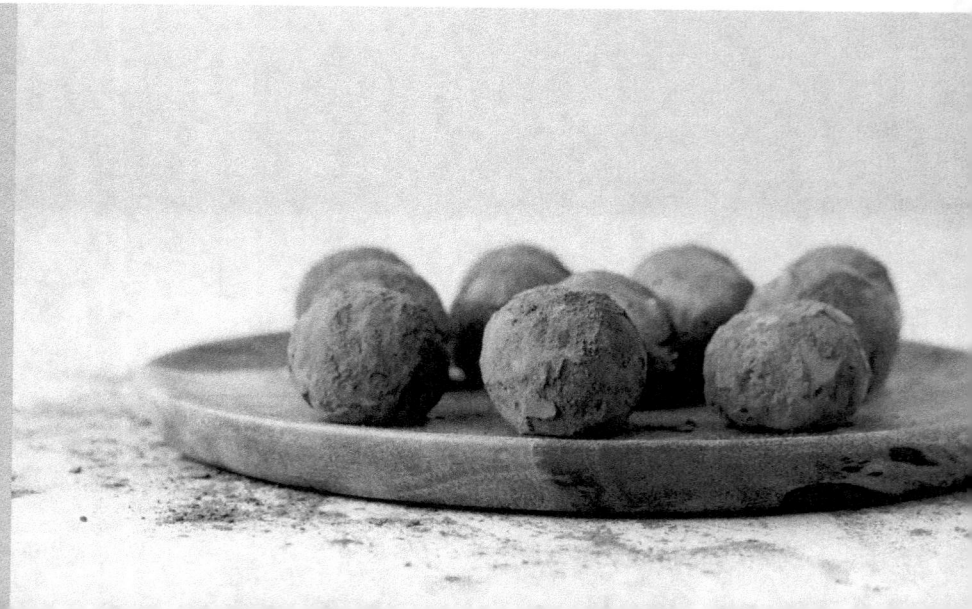

Lunch

Creamy Carrot Soup

Prep Time: 10 minutes
Cook Time: 25 minutes
Serves: 4
Difficulty Level: 1
Cost: $$

SERVING SUGGESTION

SPRINKLE WITH CINNAMON IF DESIRED.

Ingredients:

- 6 carrots peeled and washed and chopped
- 1 sweet yellow onion, chopped
- 2 cloves of garlic, chopped
- 5 cups of vegetable stock
- 1 cup full-fat unsweetened coconut milk
- Sea salt & pepper to taste
- Coconut oil for cooking

Directions:

1. Start by heating a large stockpot over medium heat with coconut oil and add the carrots, onion, and garlic. Saute for about 5 minutes.

2. Add the vegetable stock and bring to a boil. Reduce heat to a simmer and cook for about 20 minutes.

3. Remove from heat and add the coconut milk and salt and pepper. Using an immersion blender, blend until smooth or blend in a blender.

4. Pour into a serving bowl and enjoy!

Nutritional Information:
Carbs: 14g
Fiber: 3g
Net Carbs: 11g
Protein: 8g
Fat: 5g
Calories: 129

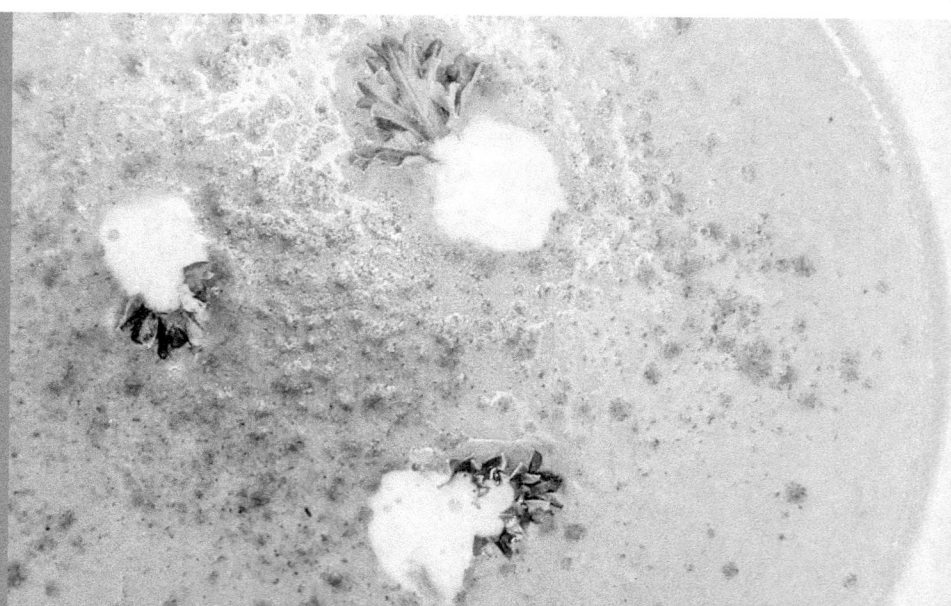

Creamy Coconut Broccoli Soup

Prep Time: 10 minutes
Cook Time: 25 minutes
Serves: 4
Difficulty Level: 1
Cost: $$

· SERVING SUGGESTION ·
ADD AN EXTRA DRIZZLE OF COCONUT MILK BEFORE SERVING IF DESIRED.

Ingredients:

- 2 cups of broccoli florets
- 1 sweet yellow onion, chopped
- 2 cloves of garlic, chopped
- 5 cups chicken broth
- 1 cup full-fat unsweetened coconut milk
- Sea salt & pepper to taste
- Coconut oil for cooking

Directions:

1. Start by heating a large stockpot over medium heat with coconut oil and add the broccoli florets, onion, and garlic. Saute for about 5 minutes.

2. Add the chicken broth and bring to a boil. Reduce heat to a simmer and cook for about 20 minutes.

3. Remove from heat and add the coconut milk and salt and pepper. Using an immersion blender, blend until smooth or blend in a blender.

4. Pour into a serving bowl and enjoy!

Nutritional Information:
Carbs: 8g
Fiber: 2g
Net Carbs: 6g
Protein: 8g
Fat: 5g
Calories: 107

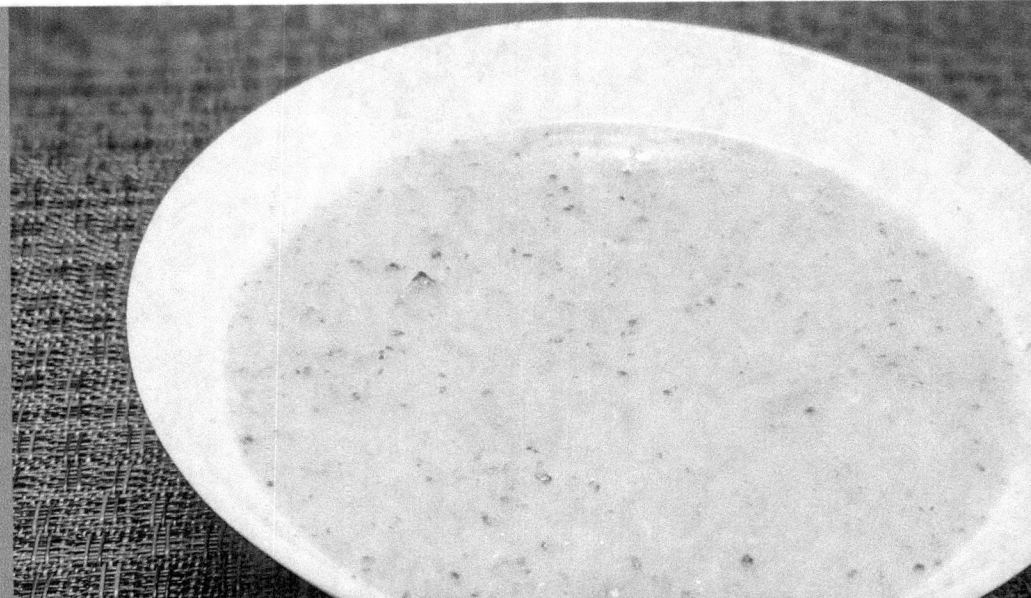

Roasted Garlic & Broccoli Soup

Prep Time: 10 minutes
Cook Time: 25 minutes
Serves: 4
Difficulty Level: 1
Cost: $$

Ingredients:

- 2 cups of broccoli florets
- 1 sweet yellow onion, chopped
- 1 head of garlic, roasted
- 5 cups chicken broth
- 1 cup full-fat unsweetened coconut milk 1 bay leaf
- Sea salt & pepper to taste
- Coconut oil for cooking

Directions:

1. Start by heating a large stockpot over medium heat with coconut oil and add the broccoli florets, and onion. Saute for about 5 minutes.

2. Add the chicken broth and the roasted garlic cloves and bay leaf. Bring to a boil. Reduce heat to a simmer and cook for about 20 minutes.

3. Remove from heat and remove the bay leaf. Add the coconut milk and salt and pepper. Using an immersion blender, blend until smooth or blend in a blender.

4. Pour into a serving bowl and enjoy!

SERVING SUGGESTION
ADD AN EXTRA DRIZZLE OF COCONUT MILK, A SPRINKLE OF CAYENNE PEPPER AND BLACK SESAME SEEDS IF DESIRED.

Nutritional Information:
Carbs: 10g
Fiber: 2g
Net Carbs: 8g
Protein: 8g
Fat: 5g
Calories: 116

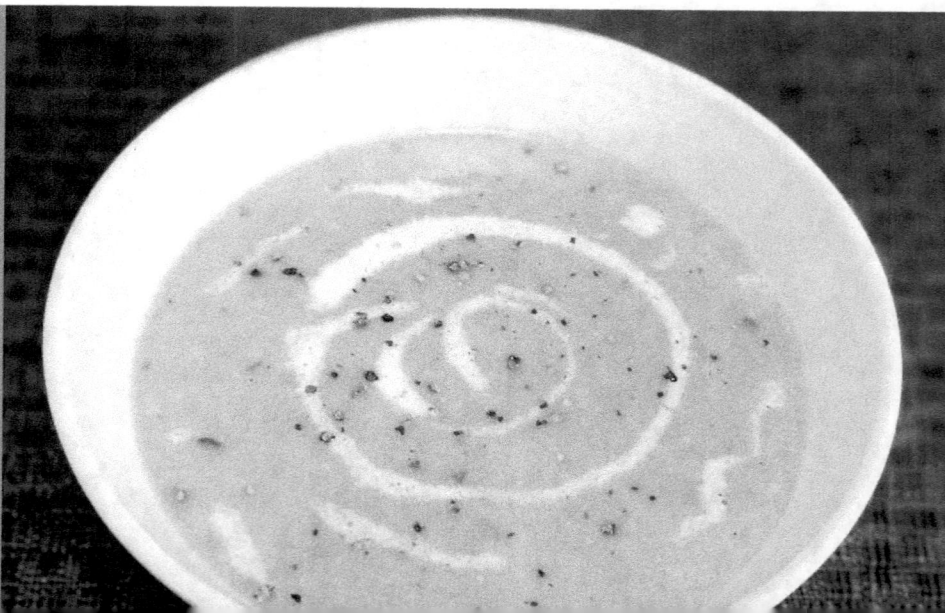

Simple Tomato Soup

Prep Time: 10 minutes
Cook Time: 25 minutes
Serves: 4
Difficulty Level: 1
Cost: $$

Ingredients:

- 2 cloves of garlic, chopped
- 1 yellow onion, chopped
- 1 (14.5 ounce) can of diced tomatoes
- 3 cups of chicken broth
- 1 tbsp fresh rosemary, chopped
- 1 cup full-fat unsweetened coconut milk
- Sea salt & pepper to taste
- Coconut oil for cooking

Directions:

1. Start by heating a large stockpot over medium heat with coconut oil and add the garlic and onion. Saute for about 5 minutes.

2. Add the diced tomatoes, chicken broth, and rosemary and bring to a boil. Reduce heat to a simmer and cook for about 20 minutes.

3. Remove from heat add the coconut milk and salt and pepper. Using an immersion blender, blend until smooth or blend in a blender.

4. Pour into a serving bowl and enjoy!

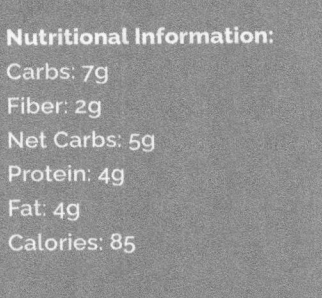

SERVING SUGGESTION

ADD AN EXTRA DRIZZLE OF COCONUT MILK IF DESIRED.

Nutritional Information:
Carbs: 7g
Fiber: 2g
Net Carbs: 5g
Protein: 4g
Fat: 4g
Calories: 85

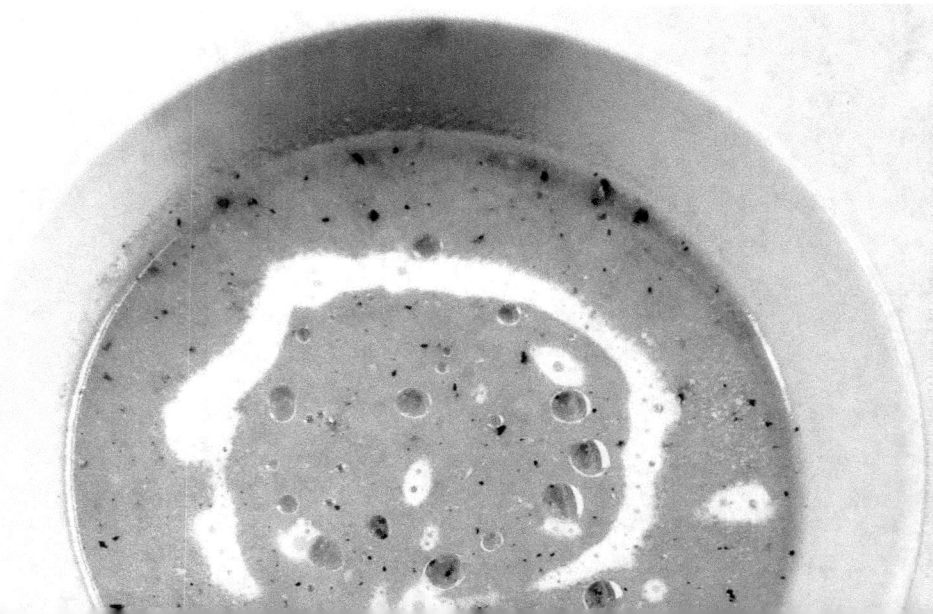

Leek & Onion Soup

Prep Time: 10 minutes
Cook Time: 25 minutes
Serves: 4
Difficulty Level: 1
Cost: $$

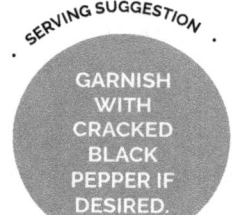

• SERVING SUGGESTION •

GARNISH WITH CRACKED BLACK PEPPER IF DESIRED.

Ingredients:

- 2 cloves of garlic, chopped
- 1 shallot, chopped
- 1 leek washed and chopped
- 4 cups of chicken broth
- 1 tbsp fresh thyme, chopped
- 1 bay leaf
- 1 cup full-fat unsweetened coconut milk
- Sea salt & pepper to taste
- Coconut oil for cooking

Directions:

1. Start by heating a large stockpot over medium heat with coconut oil and add the garlic, shallot, and leek. Saute for about 5 minutes.

2. Add the chicken broth, thyme, and bay leaf, and bring to a boil. Reduce heat to a simmer and cook for about 20 minutes.

3. Remove from heat, remove the bay leaf, add the coconut milk and salt and pepper. Using an immersion blender, blend until smooth or blend in a blender.

4. Pour into a serving bowl and enjoy!

Nutritional Information:
Carbs: 6g
Fiber: 1g
Net Carbs: 5g
Protein: 6g
Fat: 5g
Calories: 90

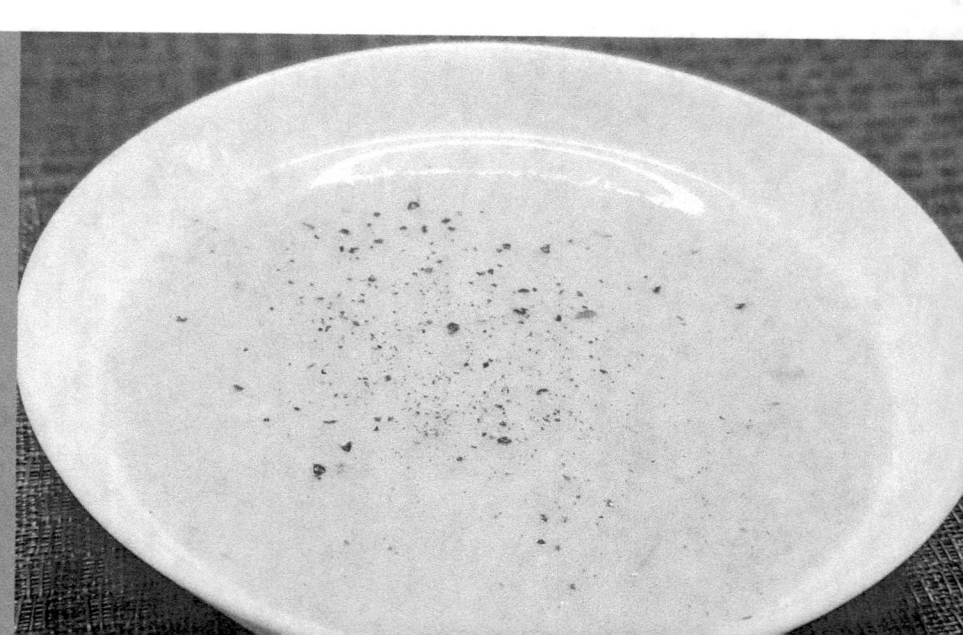

Egg Over Easy With Peppers & Onions

Prep Time: 10 minutes
Cook Time: 25 minutes
Serves: 2
Difficulty Level: 1
Cost: $$

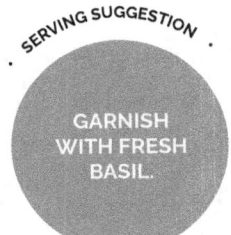

SERVING SUGGESTION

GARNISH WITH FRESH BASIL.

Ingredients:

- ½ red bell pepper, chopped
- ¼ red onion, chopped
- ½ cup broccoli florets
- 2 chicken sausages, cooked
- and sliced
- 2 eggs
- Coconut oil for cooking

Directions:

1. Start by heating a large skillet over medium heat with coconut oil. Add the bell pepper, onion, broccoli, and chicken sausage and cook for about 7minutes or until the veggies are tender.

2. Crack the eggs into the pan and cook to your liking.

3. Enjoy!

Nutritional Information:
Carbs: 11g
Fiber: 1g
Net Carbs: 10g
Protein: 18g
Fat: 17g
Calories: 264

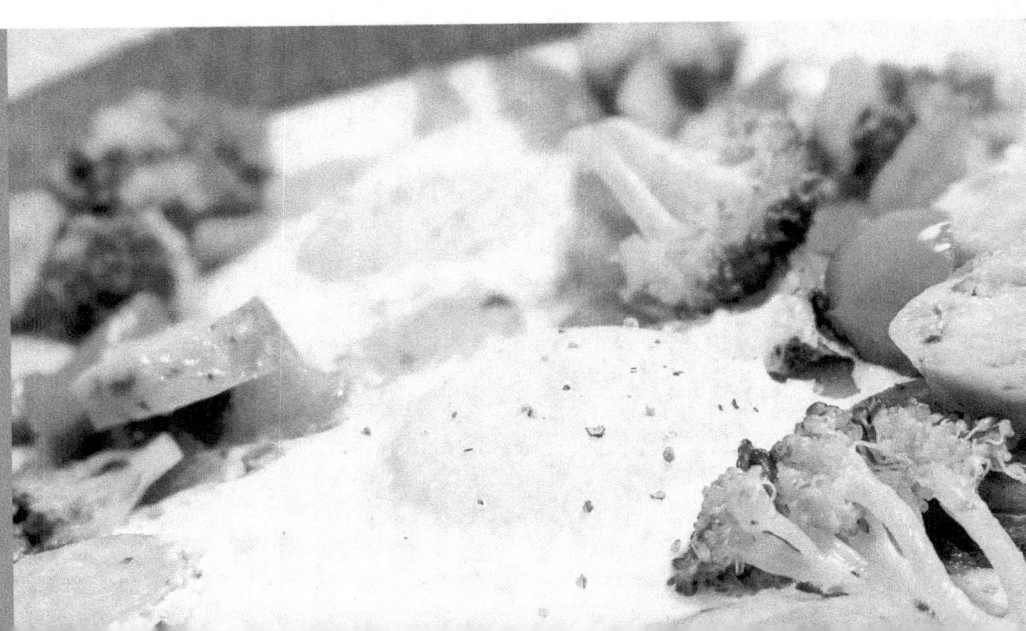

Egg "Pizza"

Prep Time: 5 minutes
Cook Time: 7 minutes
Serves: 3
Difficulty Level: 1
Cost: $$

Ingredients:

- 3 eggs
- 1 clove of garlic, chopped
- 1 red onion, thinly sliced
- 4 cherry tomatoes, halved
- 1 tbsp fresh parsley, chopped
- ½ tsp sea salt
- 1 avocado, sliced for serving
- Coconut oil for cooking

Directions::

1. Start by heating a medium skillet over medium heat with the coconut oil.

2. Add the eggs to a mixing bowl and whisk well.

3. Pour the eggs onto the skillet and add the onion, tomatoes, and parsley.

4. Cook for about 7 minutes or until the eggs are cooked and set.

5. Serve with sliced avocado.

6. Enjoy!

. SERVING SUGGESTION .

SERVE WITH MARINARA SAUCE FOR ADDED PIZZA FLAVOR!

Nutritional Information:
Carbs: 16g
Fiber: 7g
Net Carbs: 9g
Protein: 9g
Fat: 18g
Calories: 246

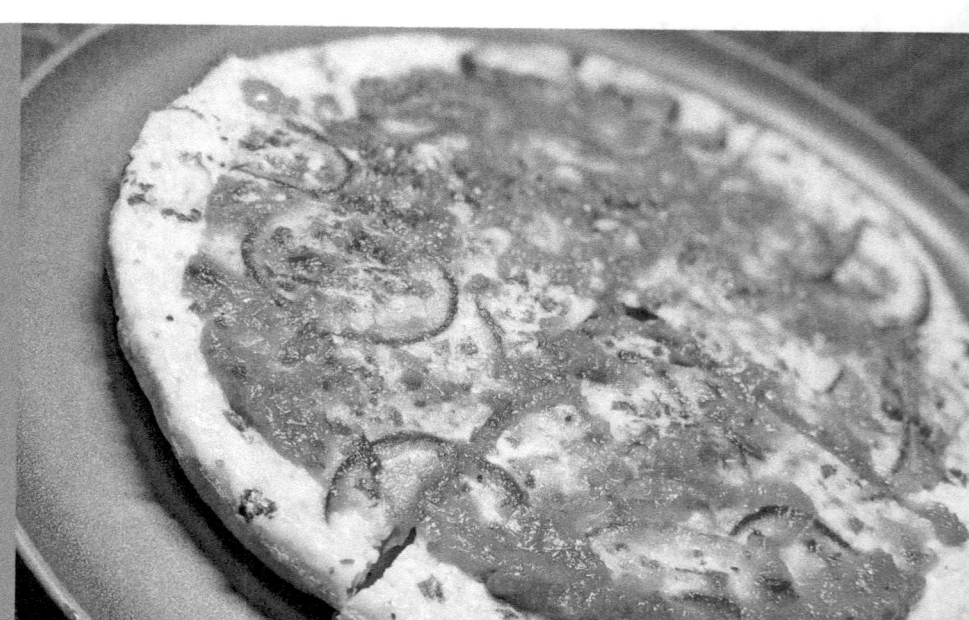

Beef Stuffed Peppers

Prep Time: 15 minutes
Cook Time: 15-20minutes
Serves: 6
Difficulty Level: 2
Cost: $$

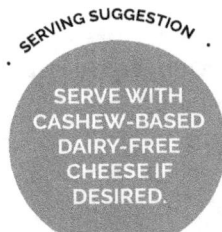

SERVING SUGGESTION

SERVE WITH CASHEW-BASED DAIRY-FREE CHEESE IF DESIRED.

Ingredients:

- 1 lb ground beef, cooked
- 2 cloves of garlic, chopped
- 1 yellow onion, chopped
- ¼ cup corn
- 1 tsp cumin
- 1 tsp oregano
- 1 tsp sea salt
- 1 red bell pepper seeded and halved
- 1 orange bell pepper seeded and halved
- 1 green bell pepper seeded and halved
- Fresh cilantro for serving
- 2 avocados, sliced for serving

Directions:

1. Start by preheating the oven to 350 degrees F and line a baking sheet with parchment paper.

2. Add the cooked ground beef, garlic, onion, corn, cumin, oregano, and salt to a mixing bowl and mix well.

3. Scoop into each bell pepper half.

4. Bake for 15-20 minutes.

5. Garnish with fresh cilantro and serve with fresh avocado.

6. Enjoy!

Nutritional Information:
Carbs: 10g
Fiber: 6g
Net Carbs: 4g
Protein: 25g
Fat: 18g
Calories: 298

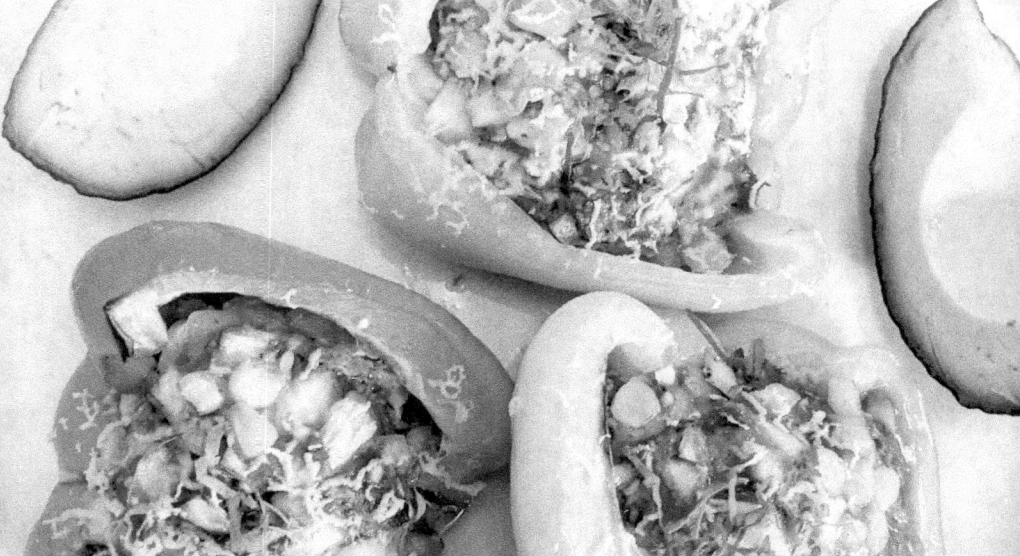

Garlic & Herb Zucchini Shrimp Scampi

Prep Time: 10 minutes
Cook Time: 3-5 minutes
Serves: 2
Difficulty Level: 2
Cost: $$

Ingredients:

- 8 shrimp, cooked
- 2 zucchinis, spiralized
- 4 tbsp olive oil
- 2 cloves of garlic, chopped
- 1 tbsp shallot, chopped
- 1 tsp onion powder
- 1 tsp Italian seasoning
- 2 cherry tomatoes, halved

Directions:

1. Start by adding the spiralized zucchini to a skillet with the olive oil and remaining ingredients. Mix well and cook for about 3-5 minutes.

2. Serve with cooked shrimp.

3. Enjoy!

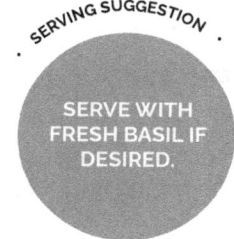

· SERVING SUGGESTION ·

SERVE WITH FRESH BASIL IF DESIRED.

Nutritional Information:
Carbs: 15g
Fiber: 3g
Net Carbs: 12g
Protein: 24g
Fat: 31g
Calories: 415

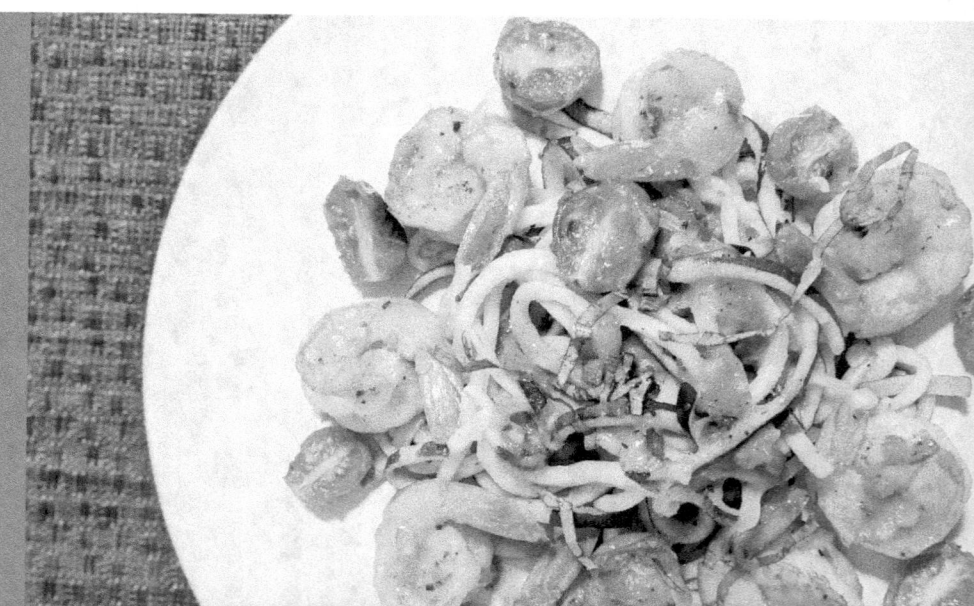

Protein-Packed Supergreens Tuna Salad

Prep Time: 10 minutes
Cook Time: 0 minutes
Serves: 2
Difficulty Level: 1
Cost: $$

Ingredients:

- 1 cup romaine lettuce
- 1 can of tuna
- 1 small red onion, thinly sliced
- 2 hard-boiled eggs
- 1 avocado, sliced
- 1 red bell pepper, seeded and sliced
- 1 tbsp olive oil
- 1 tbsp balsamic vinegar
- Sea salt & pepper to taste

Directions:

1. Assemble the salad by adding the lettuce to the base of a serving plate and top with the tuna, red onion, hard-boiled egg, avocado, and bell pepper.

2. Drizzle with olive oil and balsamic vinegar.

3. Season with salt and pepper.

4. Enjoy!

SERVING SUGGESTION

SERVE WITH ARUGULA IN PLACE OF LETTUCE IF DESIRED.

Nutritional Information:

Carbs: 15g
Fiber: 8g
Net Carbs: 7g
Protein: 32g
Fat: 38g
Calories: 521

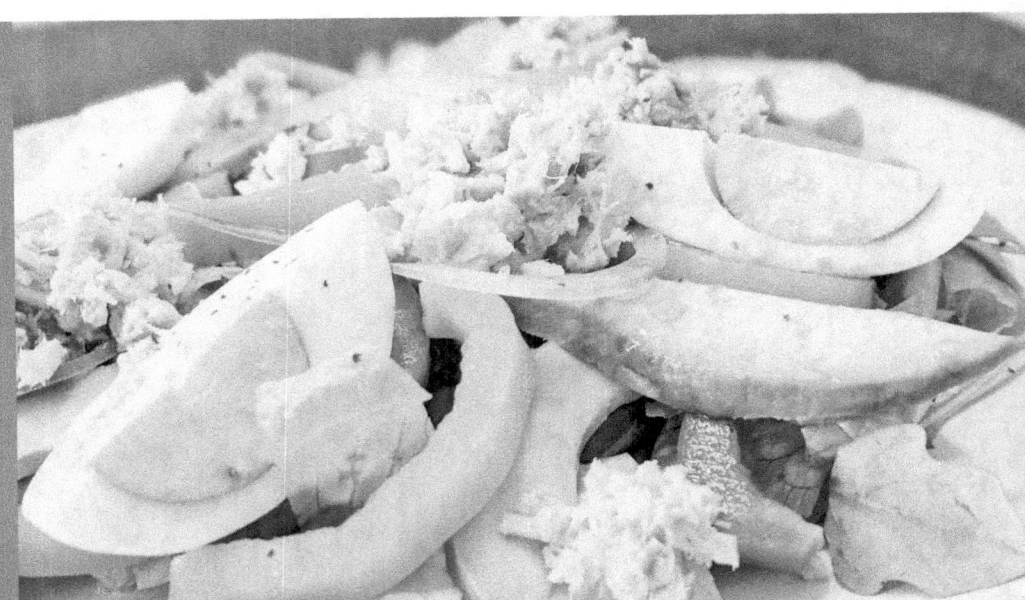

Kale Cesar Salad

Prep Time: 10 minutes
Cook Time: 0 minutes
Serves: 2
Difficulty Level: 1
Cost: $$

Ingredients:

- 2 cups romaine lettuce
- 1 avocado, cubed
- ¼ cup slivered almonds
- 1 tbsp olive oil
- 1 tbsp freshly squeezed lemon juice
- 1 tsp dijon mustard
- ½ tsp garlic powder
- Sea salt & pepper to taste

Directions:

1. Assemble the salad by adding the lettuce to the base of a serving plate and top with the avocado, and almonds.
2. Add the olive oil, lemon juice, dijon mustard, garlic powder, salt, and pepper to a mixing bowl and whisk.
3. Drizzle the dressing over the salad.
4. Enjoy!

SERVING SUGGESTION

SERVE WITH ROTISSERIE CHICKEN FOR ADDED PROTEIN IF DESIRED.

Nutritional Information:
Carbs: 14g
Fiber: 9g
Net Carbs: 5g
Protein: 5g
Fat: 33g
Calories: 347

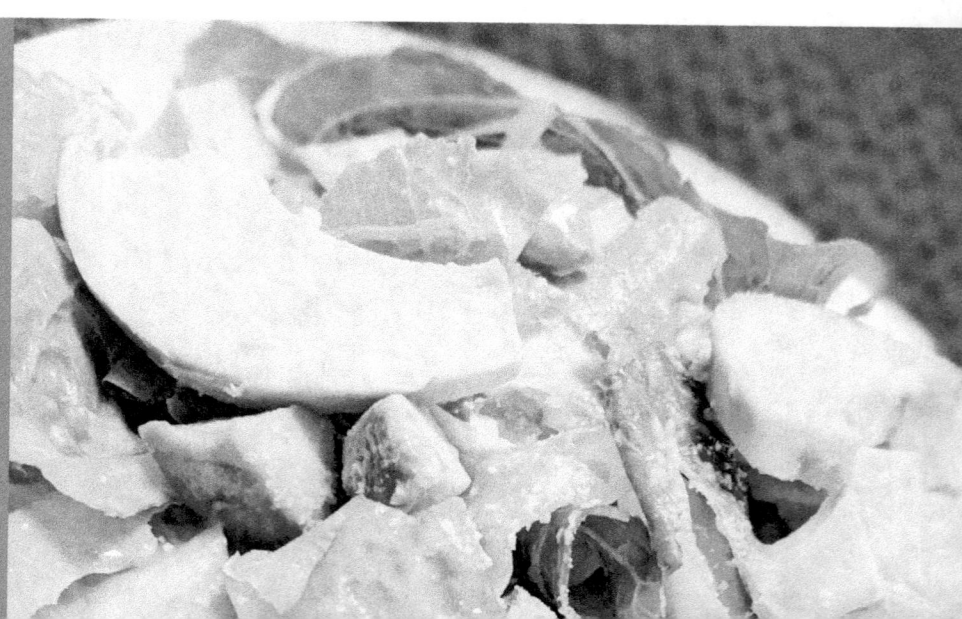

Protein Powered Salad Bowl

Prep Time: 10 minutes
Cook Time: 0 minutes
Serves: 2
Difficulty Level: 1
Cost: $$

Ingredients:

- 2 cups arugula
- 1 hard-boiled egg
- 1 red bell pepper, seeded and sliced
- 3 cherry heirloom tomatoes, halved
- 2 tbsp almonds
- 2 tbsp olive oil
- 1 tbsp balsamic vinegar
- 1 avocado, sliced

Directions:

1. Assemble the salad by adding the lettuce to the base of a serving plate and top with the avocado, and almonds.
2. Add the olive oil, lemon juice, dijon mustard, garlic powder, salt, and pepper to a mixing bowl and whisk.
3. Drizzle the dressing over the salad.
4. Enjoy!

SERVING SUGGESTION

SERVE WITH NUT AND SEED CRACKERS IF DESIRED.

Nutritional Information:
Carbs: 16g
Fiber: 9g
Net Carbs: 7g
Protein: 8g
Fat: 39g
Calories: 420

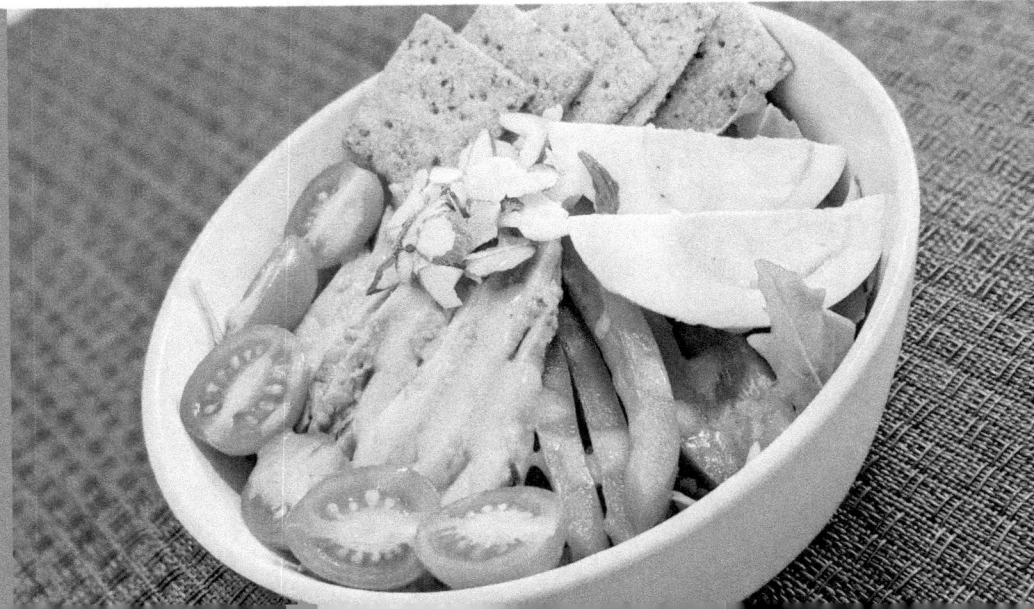

Snacks

Toasted Shredded Coconut

Prep Time: 10 minutes
Cook Time: 5 minutes
Serves: 18
Difficulty Level: 1
Cost: $$

SERVING SUGGESTION

MIX INTO HOMEMADE TRAIL MIX FOR AN ADDED BOOST OF FAT AND FLAVOR!

Ingredients:

- 3 cups shredded unsweetened coconut

Directions:

1. Simply preheat a large skillet over low to medium heat.
2. Add the shredded coconut and toast for about 5 minutes, stirring frequently.
3. Enjoy as a tasty snack or dairy-free yogurt topper!

Nutritional Information:
Carbs: 2g
Fiber: 1g
Net Carbs: 1g
Protein: 1g
Fat: 5g
Calories: 47

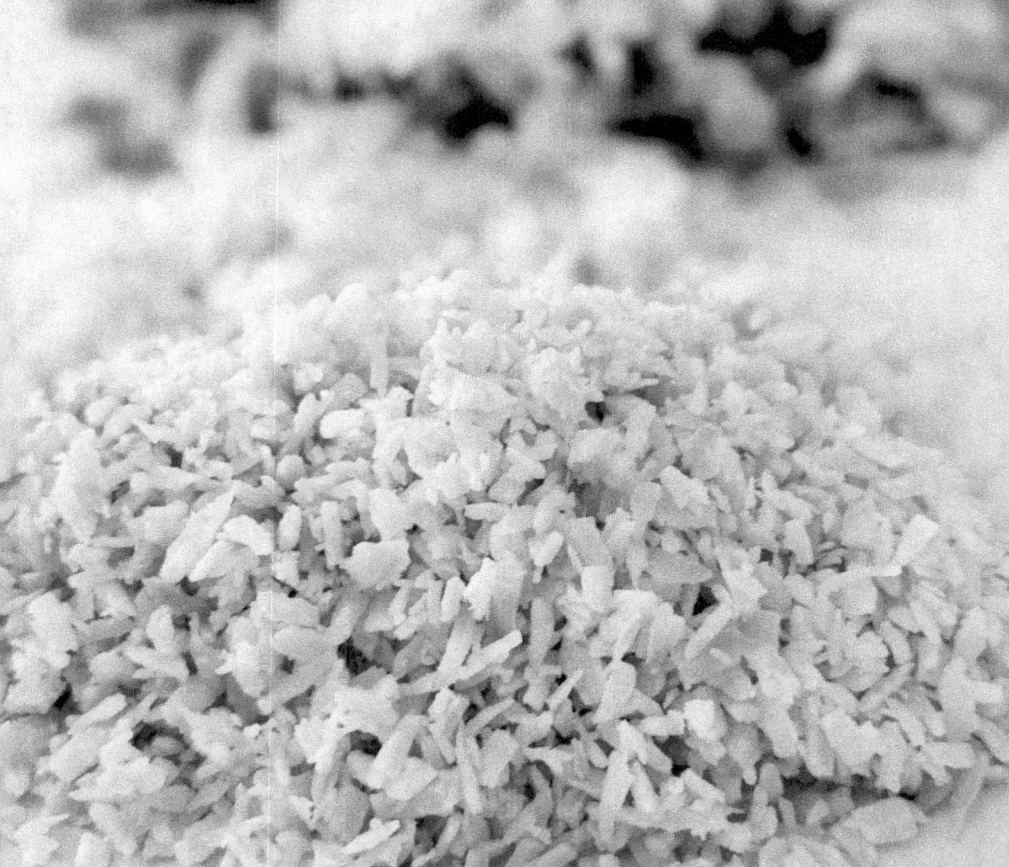

Simple Toasted Almonds

Prep Time: 10 minutes
Cook Time: 7-10 minutes
Serves: 10
Difficulty Level: 1
Cost: $$

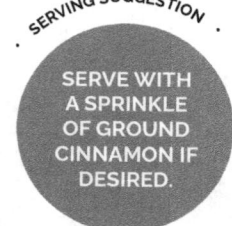

SERVING SUGGESTION

SERVE WITH A SPRINKLE OF GROUND CINNAMON IF DESIRED.

Ingredients:

- 2 cups whole raw almonds
- Pinch of sea salt

Directions:

1. Start by preheating the oven to 300 degrees F and line a baking sheet with parchment paper.

2. Add the raw almonds to a single layer to the baking sheet and bake for about 7-10 minutes, checking at the five minute mark as they tend to toast up quickly!

3. Serve with a sprinkle of sea salt.

Nutritional Information:
Carbs: 6g
Fiber: 4g
Net Carbs: 2g
Protein: 6g
Fat: 14g
Calories: 164

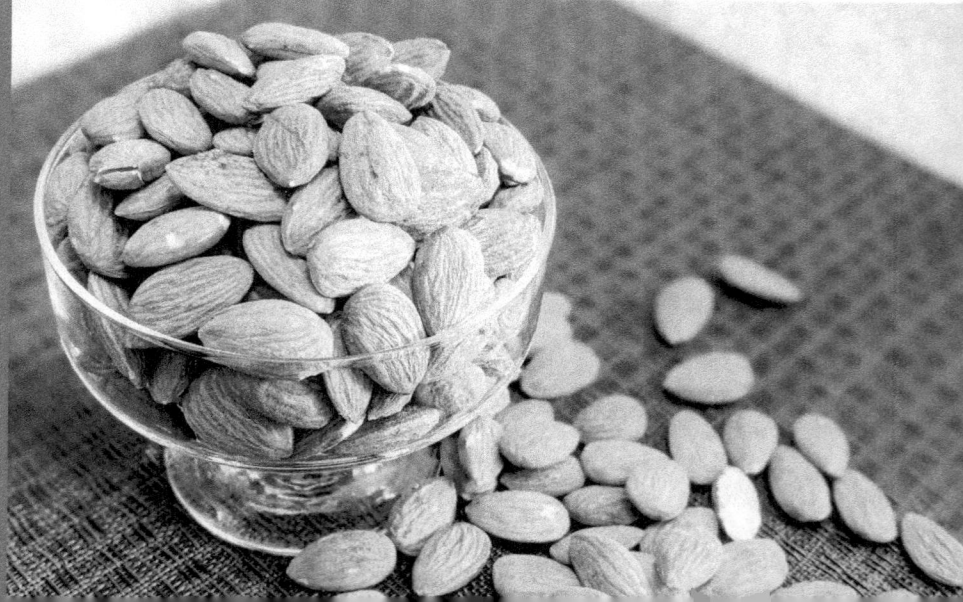

Homemade Cinnamon Almond Butter

Prep Time: 20 minutes

Cook Time: 0 minutes

Serves: 16

Difficulty Level: 2

Cost: $$

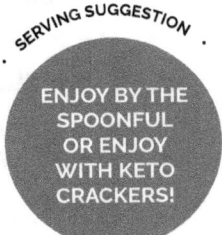

SERVING SUGGESTION

ENJOY BY THE SPOONFUL OR ENJOY WITH KETO CRACKERS!

Ingredients:

- 3 cups whole toasted almonds
- 1 tsp sea salt
- 2 tsp ground cinnamon
- 1 tsp pure vanilla extract

Directions:

1. Add the almonds to the base of a food processor and process until an almond butter consistency forms, scraping down the sides of the food processor as needed. This will take about 20 minutes.

2. Add the sea salt, cinnamon, and vanilla extract and process for another 30 seconds.

3. Store in an airtight container in the fridge.

Nutritional Information:

Carbs: 4g

Fiber: 2g

Net Carbs: 2g

Protein: 4g

Fat: 9g

Calories: 105

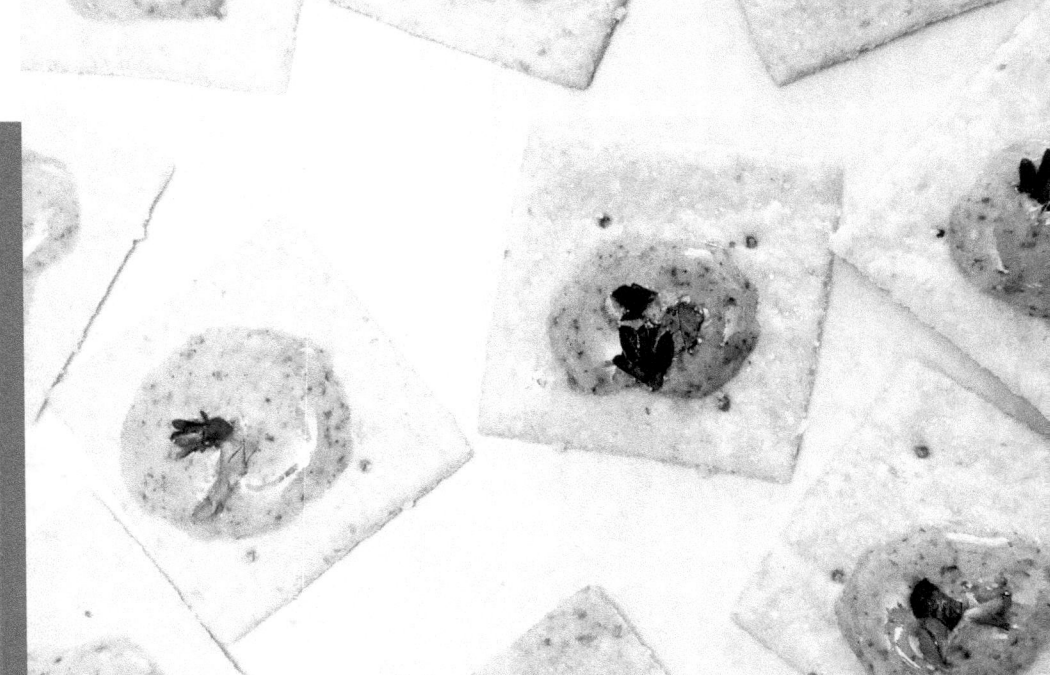

Sea Salt Vanilla Cashew Butter

Prep Time: 20 minutes
Cook Time: 0 minutes
Serves: 20
Difficulty Level: 2
Cost: $$

SERVING SUGGESTION

ENJOY BY THE SPOONFUL OR ENJOY WITH KETO CRACKERS OR BLENDED INTO LOW CARB SMOOTHIES.

Ingredients:

- 3 cups raw cashews
- 1 tsp sea salt
- 2 tsp pure vanilla extract

Directions:

1. Add the cashews to the base of a food processor and process until a cashew butter consistency forms, scraping down the sides of the food processor as needed. This will take about 20 minutes.

2. Add the sea salt and vanilla extract and process for another 30 seconds.

3. Store in an airtight container in the fridge.

Nutritional Information:

Carbs: 7g

Fiber: 1g

Net Carbs: 6g

Protein: 3g

Fat: 10g

Calories: 119

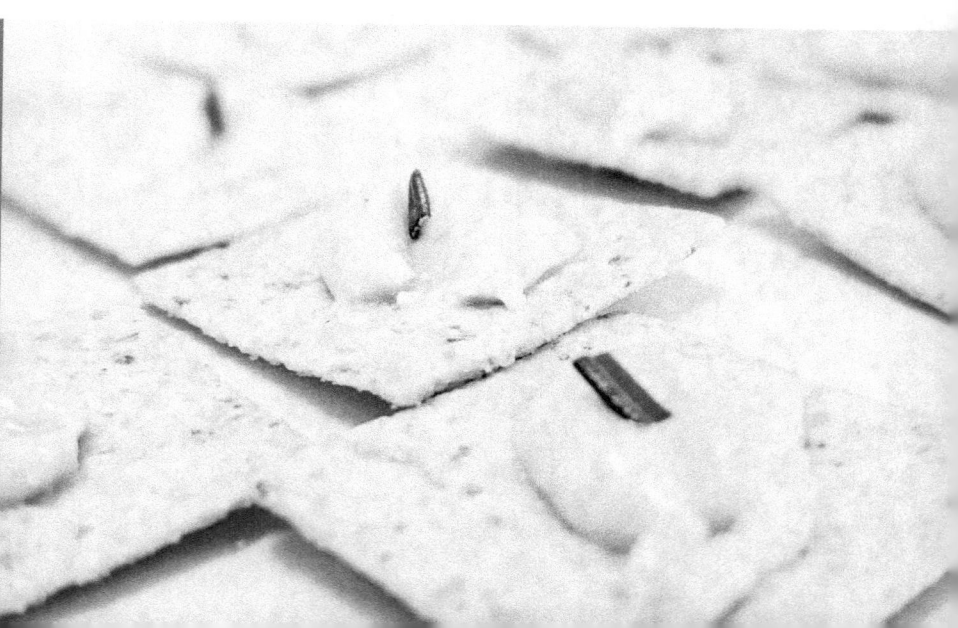

Vanilla Cake Batter Coconut Butter Bites

Prep Time: 10 minutes
+ chilling time
Cook Time: 0 minutes
Serves: 14 (1 bite per serving)
Difficulty Level: 2
Cost: $$

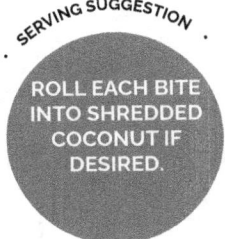

SERVING SUGGESTION

ROLL EACH BITE
INTO SHREDDED
COCONUT IF
DESIRED.

Ingredients:

- 2 cups shredded unsweetened coconut
- 2 tbsp coconut butter
- ¾ cup almond flour
- 6 drops vanilla liquid stevia
- 1 tsp sea salt
- 1 tsp pure vanilla extract
- Water

Directions:

1. Add all ingredients to a food processor or high speed blender and blend until smooth. Add a teaspoon of water at time if needed until the mixture comes together.

2. Transfer to a serving bowl and chill in the fridge for 20 minutes.

3. Once chilled, roll into bite-sized rounds.

4. Store in the fridge until ready to enjoy.

Nutritional Information:
Carbs: 3g
Fiber: 2g
Net Carbs: 1g
Protein: 1g
Fat: 7g
Calories: 76

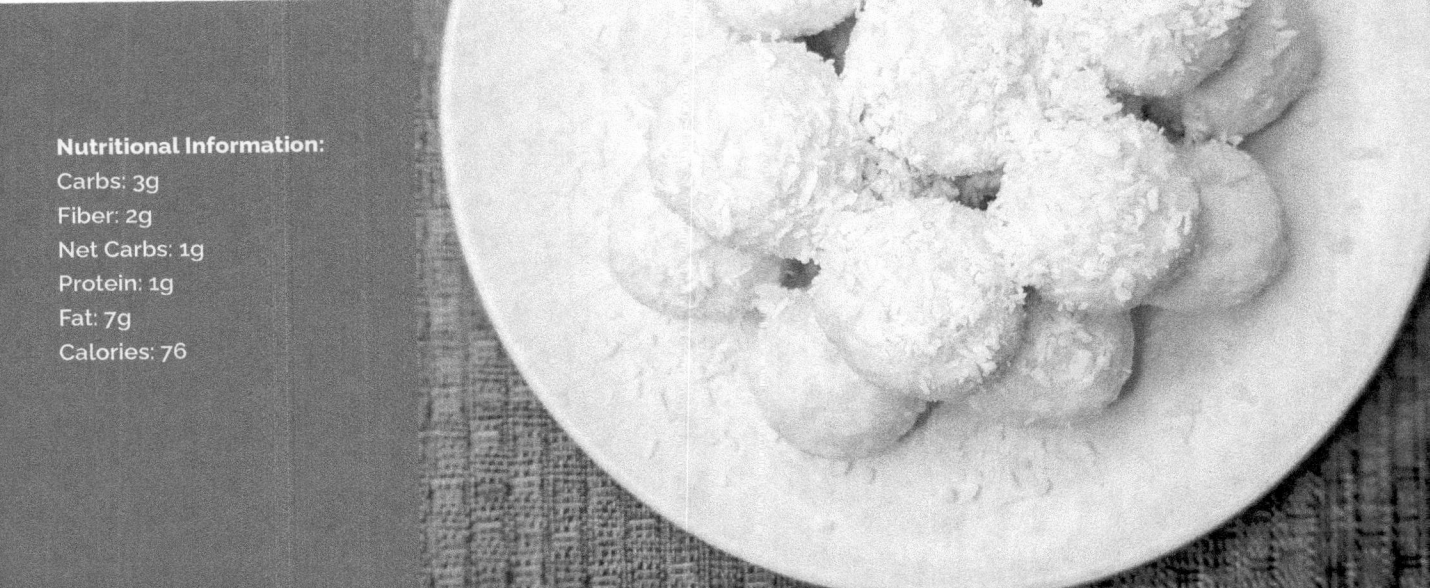

Apple Fat Bombs

Prep Time: 10 minutes
Cook Time: 0 minutes
Serves: 4
Difficulty Level: 1
Cost: $$

Ingredients:

- 1 apple, sliced
- 1 tbsp peanut butter
- 1 tbsp sugar free chocolate chips
- 1 tbsp slivered almonds
- 1 tbsp pecans, chopped

Directions:

1. Start by slicing the apples and spread with peanut butter.
2. Top with remaining toppings.
3. Enjoy!

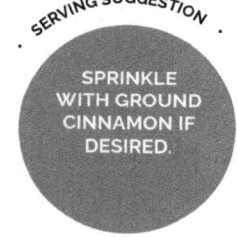

SERVING SUGGESTION

SPRINKLE WITH GROUND CINNAMON IF DESIRED.

Nutritional Information:
Carbs: 13g
Fiber: 4g
Net Carbs: 9g
Protein: 4g
Fat: 19g
Calories: 221

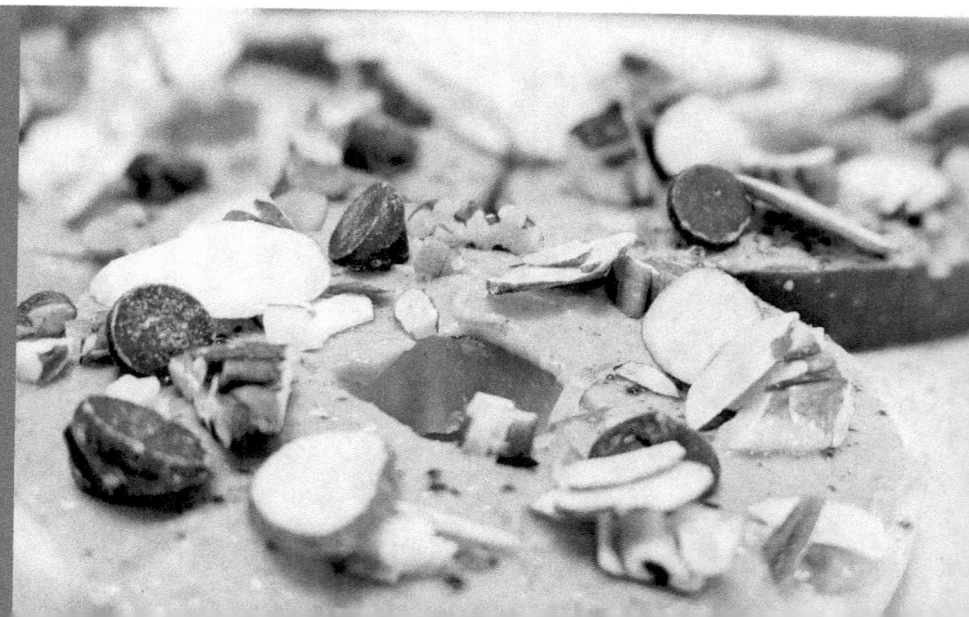

Apple Cinnamon Smoothie Snack Bowl

Prep Time: 10 minutes
Cook Time: 0 minutes
Serves: 3
Difficulty Level: 1
Cost: $

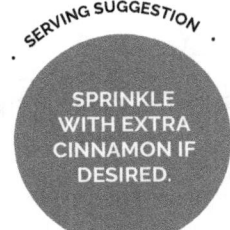

SERVING SUGGESTION

SPRINKLE WITH EXTRA CINNAMON IF DESIRED.

Ingredients:

- ½ apple, peeled and sliced
- ½ cup full fat unsweetened coconut milk
- 1 tbsp almond butter
- 1 tbsp flax seeds
- 1 tsp ground cinnamon
- **For topping:** 1 tbsp slivered almonds, ½ tbsp extra drizzle of almond butter

Directions:

1. Start by adding ½ apple, coconut milk, almond butter, and flaxseeds to a blender and blend until smooth.

2. Add to a bowl and top with the remaining apple slices, almonds, and a drizzle of almond butter.

3. Enjoy!

Nutritional Information:
Carbs: 10g
Fiber: 4g
Net Carbs: 6g
Protein: 4g
Fat: 17g
Calories: 197

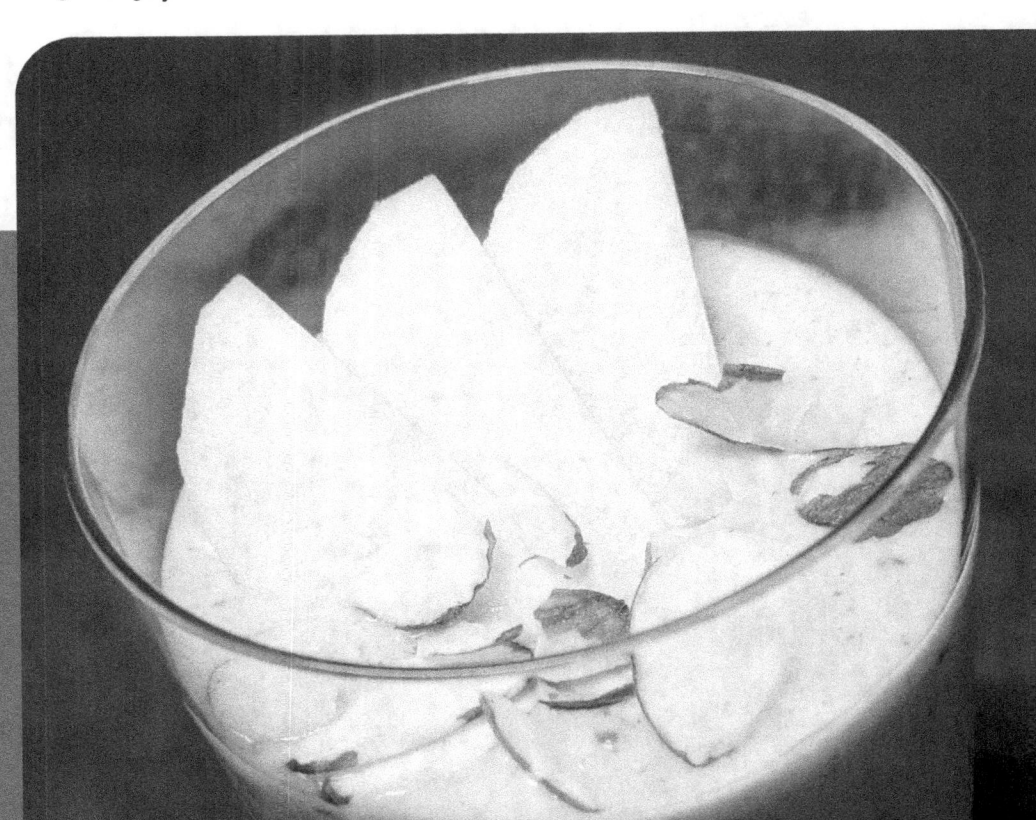

Chocolate Peanut Butter Energy Bites

Prep Time: 15 minutes
+ chilling time
Cook Time: 0 minutes
Serves: 12
Difficulty Level: 1
Cost: $$

Ingredients:

- 2 cups creamy peanut butter
- ¼ cup raw unsweetened cacao powder
- 1 tsp pure vanilla extract
- 2 tsp monk fruit sweetener

Directions:

1. Add all ingredients to a large mixing bowl and stir well until smooth.
2. Chill in the fridge for 1 hour.
3. Once chilled, roll the dough into bite-sized rounds and store in an airtight container in the fridge.

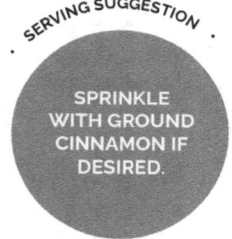

SERVING SUGGESTION

SPRINKLE WITH GROUND CINNAMON IF DESIRED.

Nutritional Information:
Carbs: 12g
Fiber: 5g
Net Carbs: 7g
Protein: 12g
Fat: 23g
Calories: 270

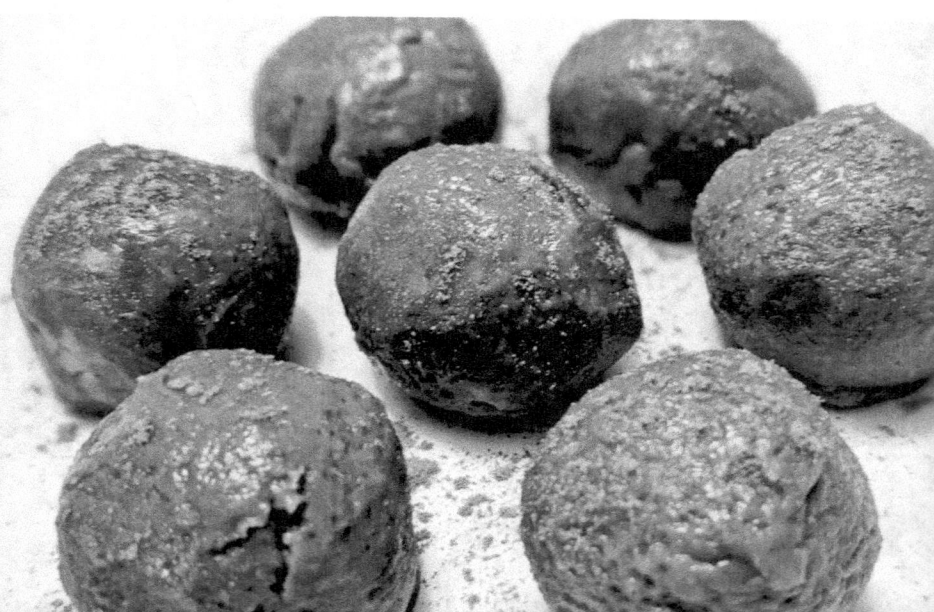

Bacon Wrapped Asparagus

Prep Time: 15 minutes
Cook Time: 20 minutes
Serves: 3
Difficulty Level: 1
Cost: $$

SERVING SUGGESTION

SPRINKLE
WITH GROUND
CINNAMON IF
DESIRED.

Ingredients:

- 21 asparagus spears
- 7 strips of bacon
- 1 tbsp coconut oil, melted

Directions:

1. Start by preheating the oven to 400 degrees F and line a baking sheet with parchment paper.

2. Add the melted coconut oil to a mixing bowl and add the asparagus spears, stir coating the spears in the oil.

3. Wrap a slice of bacon around 3 asparagus spears and place on the parchment-lined baking sheet.

4. Bake for about 20 minutes or until the bacon is crispy.

Nutritional Information:

Carbs: 7g

Fiber: 4g

Net Carbs: 3g

Protein: 20g

Fat: 23g

Calories: 312

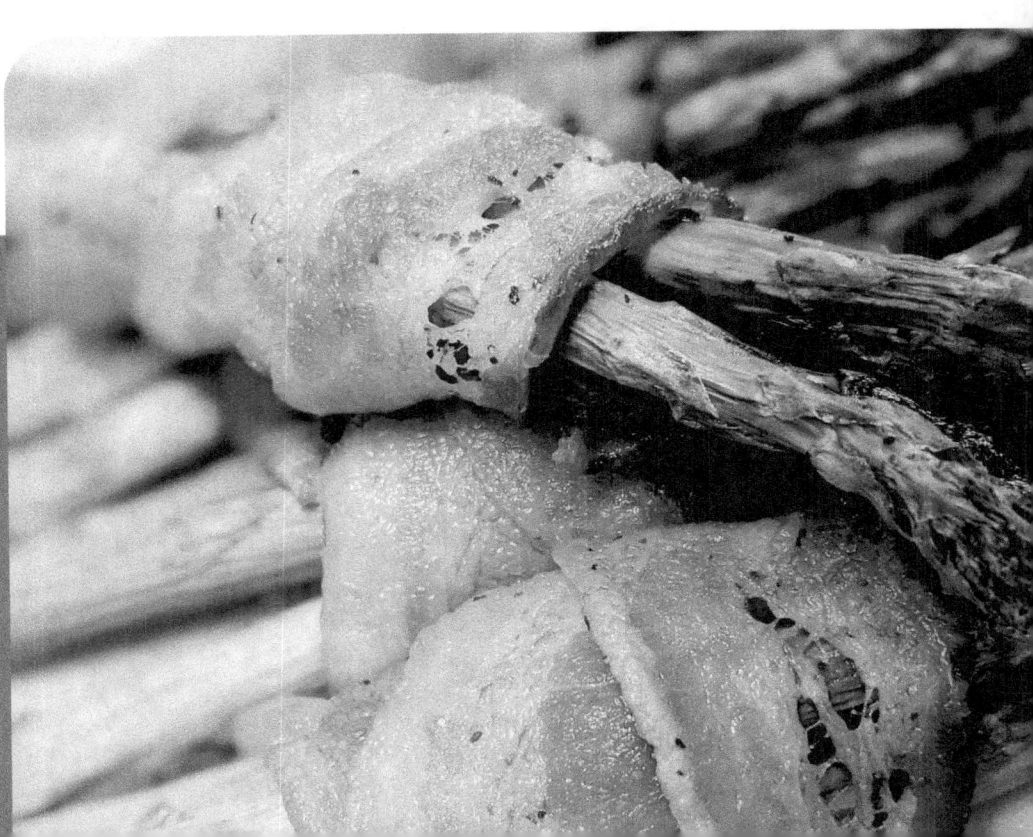

Chocolate Snack Muffins

Prep Time: 15 minutes
Cook Time: 18-20 minutes
Serves: 12
Difficulty Level: 2
Cost: $$

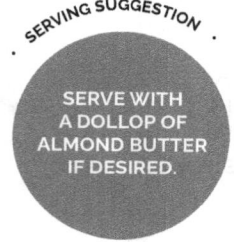

SERVING SUGGESTION

SERVE WITH A DOLLOP OF ALMOND BUTTER IF DESIRED.

Ingredients:

- 1 cup almond flour
- ½ cup erythritol
- ½ cup unsweetened cacao powder
- 1 tsp baking powder
- ½ tsp sea salt

- 2 eggs
- ¾ cup full-fat unsweetened coconut milk
- ¼ cup coconut oil, melted
- 1 tsp pure vanilla extract

Directions:

1. Start by preheating the oven to 350 degrees F and line a muffin tin with liners.

2. Add all the dry ingredients to a large mixing bowl and whisk.

3. Add the eggs to a separate mixing bowl and whisk well. Add the coconut milk, melted coconut oil, and vanilla and whisk well.

4. Add the wet ingredients to the dry and mix until smooth.

5. Pour into the lined muffin in and bake for 18-20 minutes or until a toothpick inserted into the center comes out clean.

6. Store leftovers in an airtight container in the fridge.

Nutritional Information:
Carbs: 13g
Fiber: 5g
Net Carbs: 8g
Protein: 4g
Fat: 13g
Calories: 132

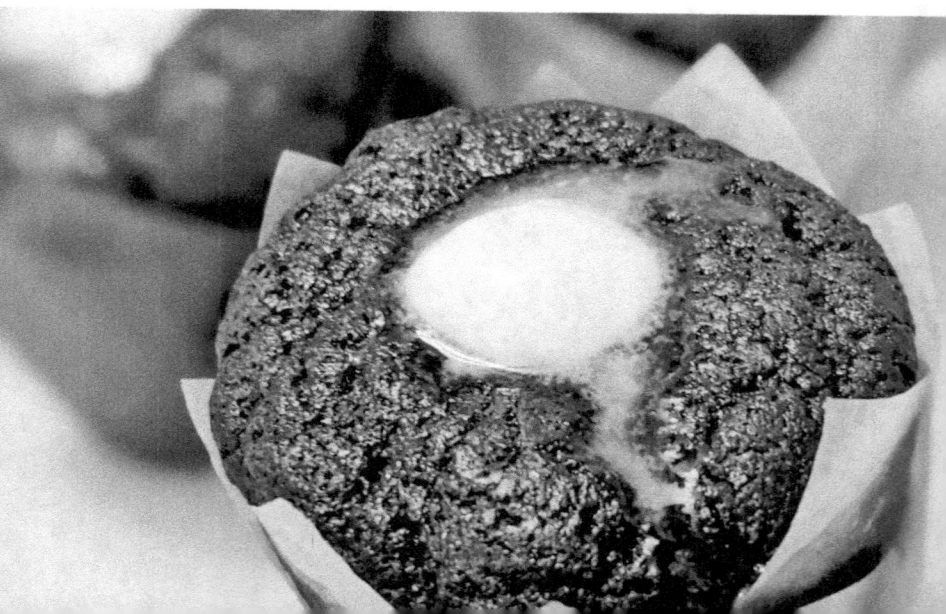

Sauteed Zucchini Rounds

Prep Time: 10 minutes
Cook Time: 4-6minutes
Serves: 2
Difficulty Level: 1
Cost: $1

Ingredients:

- 1 tbsp coconut oil
- 1 zucchini, sliced
- ½ tsp sea salt

Directions:

1. Start by heating a skillet over medium heat with the coconut oil.
2. Season the zucchini slices with salt and pepper and add to the pan.
3. Cook for about 2-3 minutes on each side or until tender.
4. Enjoy!

SERVING SUGGESTION

SERVE WITH UNSWEETENED BBQ SAUCE OR UNSWEETENED KETCHUP.

Nutritional Information:
Carbs: 3g
Fiber: 1g
Net Carbs: 2g
Protein: 1g
Fat: 7g
Calories: 74

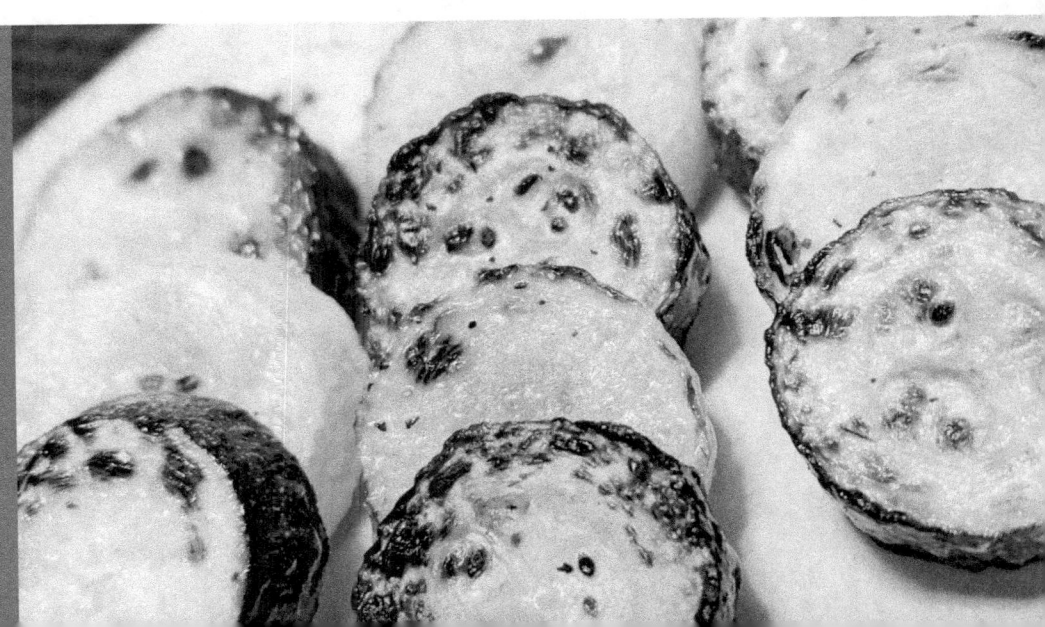

Cashew Cilantro Dip

Prep Time: 10 minutes

Cook Time: 0 minutes

Serves: 10

Difficulty Level: 1

Cost: $$

Ingredients:

- 1 cup raw cashews
- ¼ cup nutritional yeast
- ½ cup cilantro, chopped
- 2 cloves garlic, chopped
- 2 cups fire roasted diced tomatoes
- 1 tsp sea salt

Directions:

1. Add all ingredients the a blender or food processor and blend until smooth.
2. Chill in the fridge for 1 hour before serving.

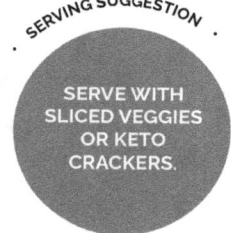

SERVING SUGGESTION

SERVE WITH SLICED VEGGIES OR KETO CRACKERS.

Nutritional Information:

Carbs: 9g

Fiber: 2g

Net Carbs: 7g

Protein: 4g

Fat: 7g

Calories: 106

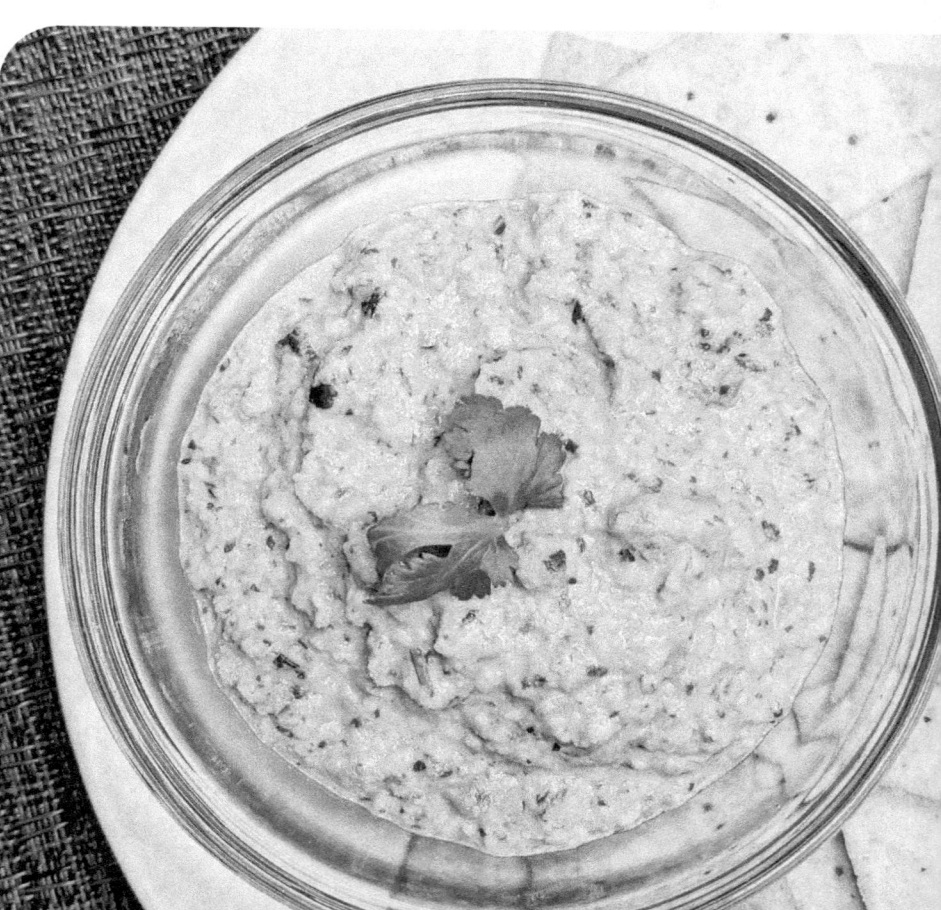

Spicy Cilantro Greens Sauce

Prep Time: 10 minutes
Cook Time: 0 minutes
Serves: 6
Difficulty Level: 1
Cost: $$

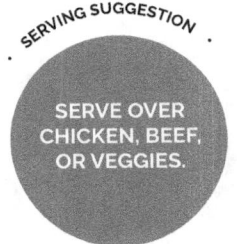

SERVING SUGGESTION

SERVE OVER CHICKEN, BEEF, OR VEGGIES.

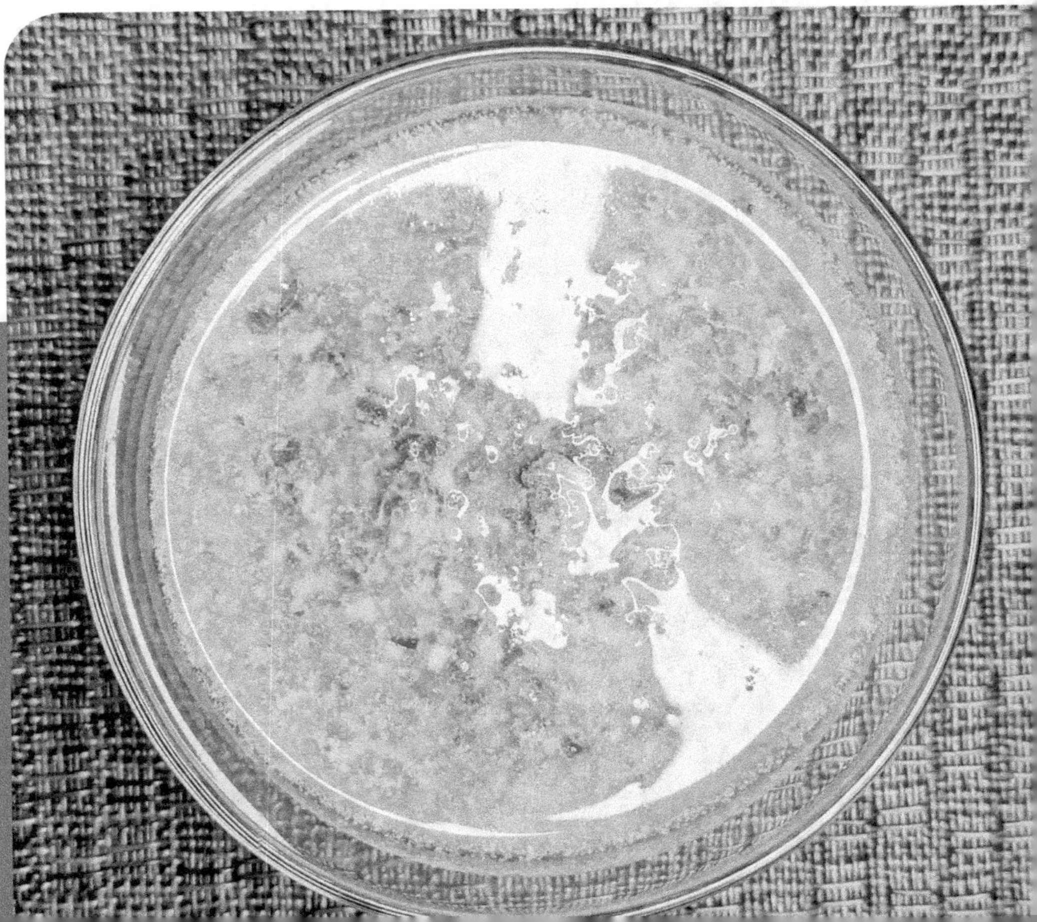

Ingredients:

- ½ cup olive oil
- ¼ cup freshly squeezed lemon juice
- ½ cup cilantro, chopped
- 1 cloves garlic, chopped
- 1 small jalapeno pepper
- 1 tsp sea salt

Directions:

1. Add all ingredients to a blender or food processor and blend until smooth.
2. Store in the fridge until ready to enjoy.

Nutritional Information:
Carbs: 1g
Fiber: 0g
Net Carbs: 1g
Protein: 0g
Fat: 17g
Calories: 148

Basil Cilantro Sauce

Prep Time: 10 minutes
Cook Time: 0 minutes
Serves: 6
Difficulty Level: 1
Cost: $$

Ingredients:

- ½ cup fresh basil
- ½ cup fresh cilantro
- 2 cloves garlic, chopped
- ¼ cup pine nuts
- ¼ cup nutritional yeast
- ¼ cup olive oil
- 1 tsp sea salt

Directions:

1. Add all ingredients to a blender or food processor and blend until smooth.
2. Store in the fridge until ready to enjoy.

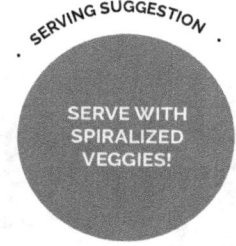

SERVING SUGGESTION

SERVE WITH SPIRALIZED VEGGIES!

Nutritional Information:
Carbs: 4g
Fiber: 2g
Net Carbs: 2g
Protein: 4g
Fat: 13g
Calories: 136

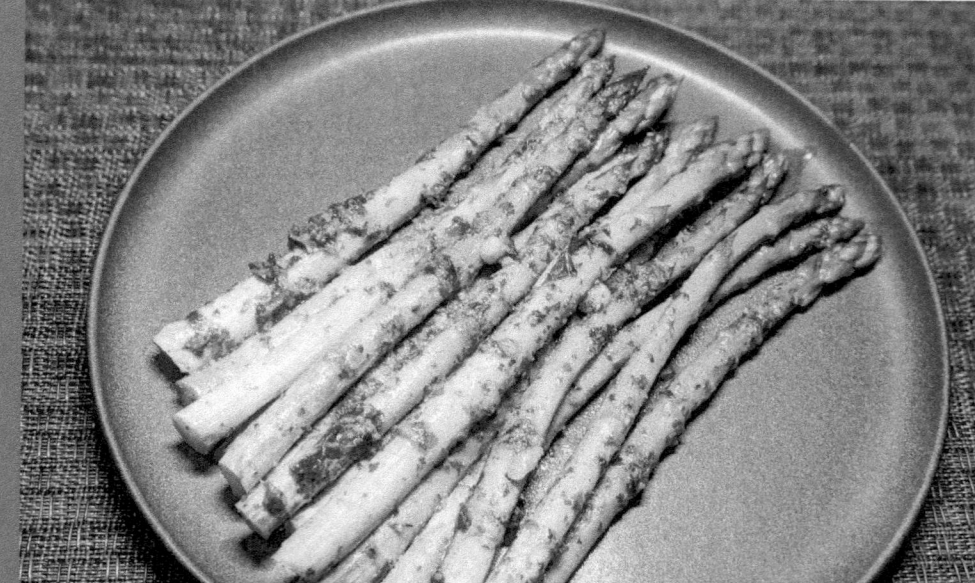

Garlic & Herb Carrots

Prep Time: 10 minutes
Cook Time: 30 minutes
Serves: 6
Difficulty Level: 1
Cost: $$

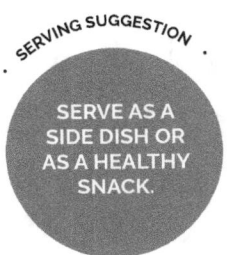

SERVING SUGGESTION

SERVE AS A SIDE DISH OR AS A HEALTHY SNACK.

Ingredients:

- 12 large carrots, washed and sliced in half lengthwise
- 2 tbsp olive oil
- 1 clove garlic, chopped
- 1 tbsp fresh rosemary, chopped
- 1 tsp sea salt
- ¼ tsp black pepper

Directions:

1. Start by preheating the oven to 375 degrees F and line a baking sheet with parchment paper.

2. Add the olive oil, garlic, rosemary, salt, and pepper to a mixing bowl and whisk.

3. Add the carrot halves to the baking sheet and drizzle with the olive oil and herb mixture.

4. Bake for 30 minutes or until tender.

5. Enjoy!

Nutritional Information:
Carbs: 15g
Fiber: 4g
Net Carbs: 11g
Protein: 1g
Fat: 5g
Calories: 102

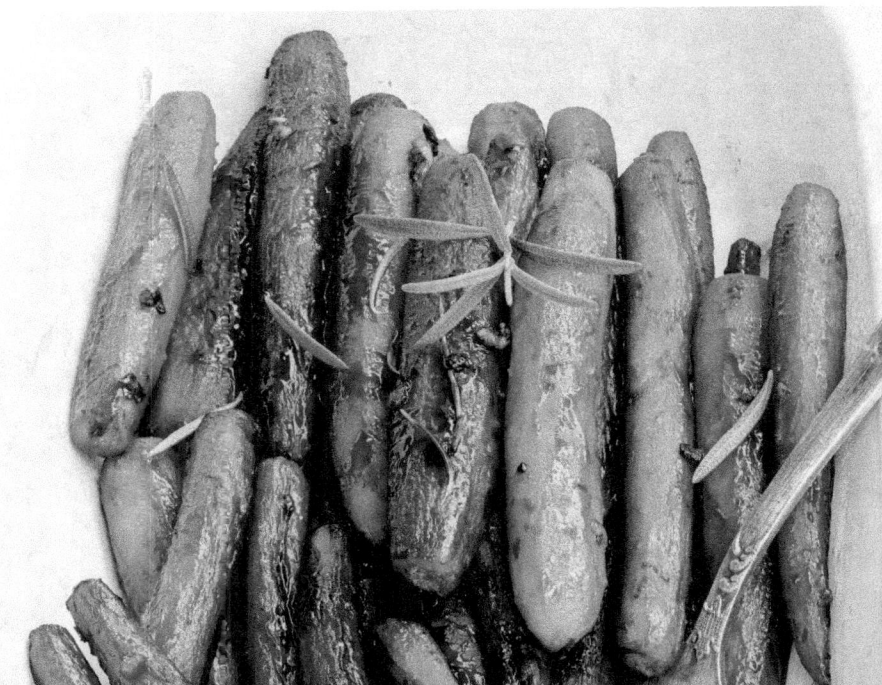

Spicy Chili Paste

Prep Time: 10 minutes
Cook Time: 0 minutes
Serves: 18
Difficulty Level: 1
Cost: $$

Ingredients:

- ½ cup olive oil
- ¼ cup tomato paste
- 1 tbsp red chili flakes
- 1 tsp onion powder
- 1 tsp garlic powder
- 1 tsp sea salt

Directions:

1. Add all ingredients to a food processor or blender and blend for 20-30 seconds.
2. Store in an airtight container in the fridge until ready to enjoy.

SERVING SUGGESTION

THIS SAUCE IS DELICIOUS WITH STIR-FRYS THAT NEED AN ADDED KICK!

Nutritional Information:

Carbs: 1g

Fiber: 0g

Net Carbs: 1g

Protein: 0g

Fat: 6g

Calories: 58

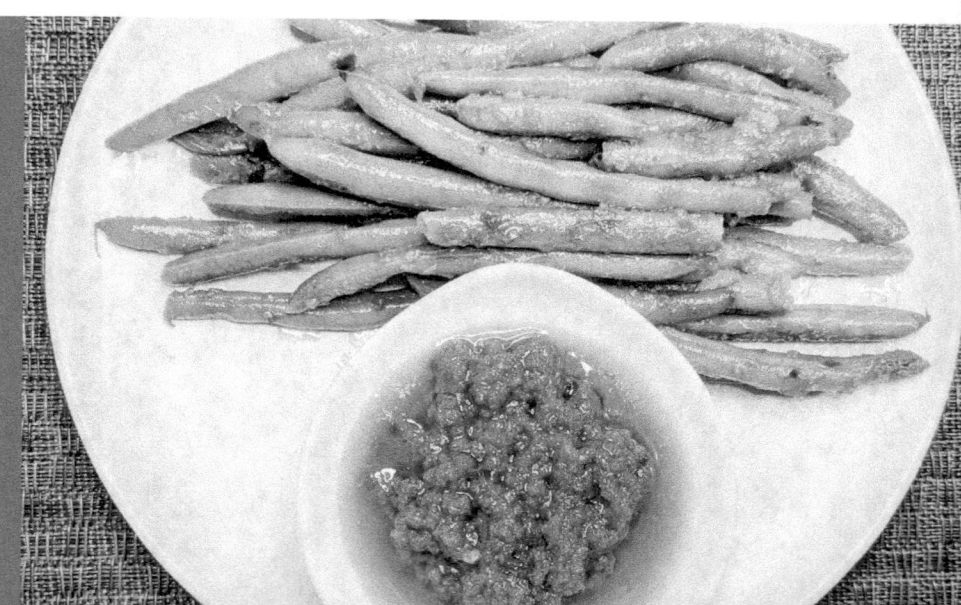

Italian Dressing

Prep Time: 10 minutes
Cook Time: 0 minutes
Serves: 10
Difficulty Level: 1
Cost: $$

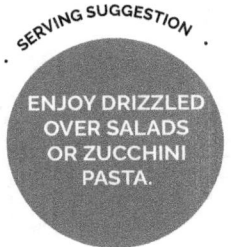

SERVING SUGGESTION

ENJOY DRIZZLED OVER SALADS OR ZUCCHINI PASTA.

Ingredients:

- 1 cup olive oil
- ½ cup white wine vinegar
- 1 tbsp Italian seasoning
- 1 tsp garlic powder
- 1 tsp oregano
- 1 tsp sea salt

Directions:

1. Add all ingredients to a jar and shake well.
2. Store in the fridge until ready to use and shake well before serving!

Nutritional Information:

Carbs: 1g

Fiber: 0g

Net Carbs: 1g

Protein: 0g

Fat: 21g

Calories: 181

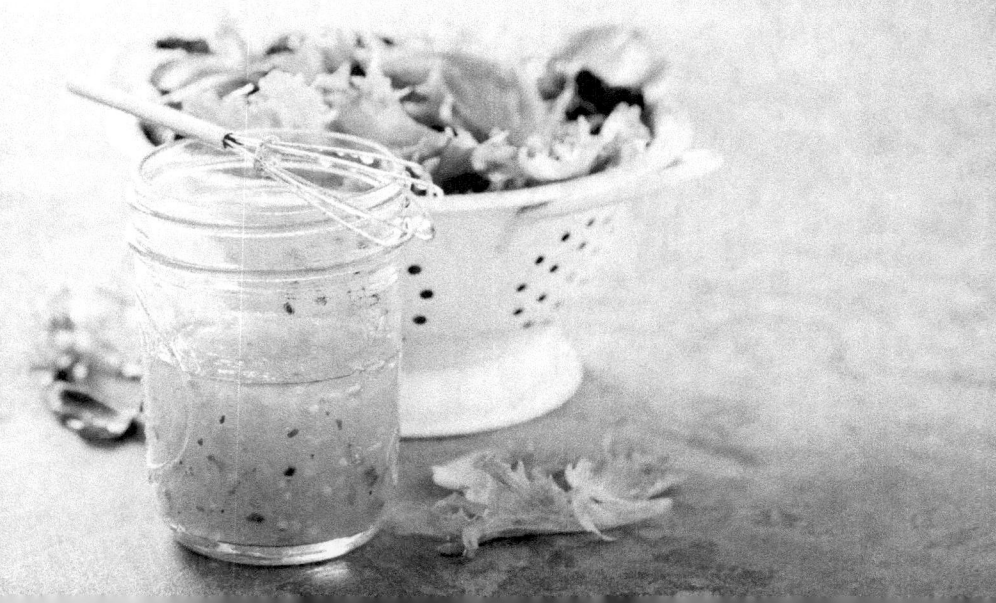

Lemon Mustard Vinaigrette

Prep Time: 10 minutes
Cook Time: 0 minutes
Serves: 10
Difficulty Level: 1
Cost: $$

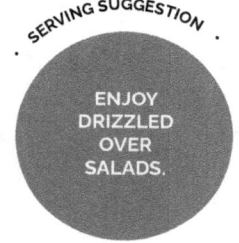

SERVING SUGGESTION

ENJOY DRIZZLED OVER SALADS.

Ingredients:

- 1 cup olive oil
- ¼ cup freshly squeezed lemon juice
- 2 tbsp dijon mustard
- 1 tsp garlic powder
- 1 tsp sea salt

Directions:

1. Add all ingredients to a jar and shake well.
2. Store in the fridge until ready to use and shake well before serving!

Nutritional Information:
Carbs: 1g
Fiber: 0g
Net Carbs: 1g
Protein: 0g
Fat: 20g
Calories: 177

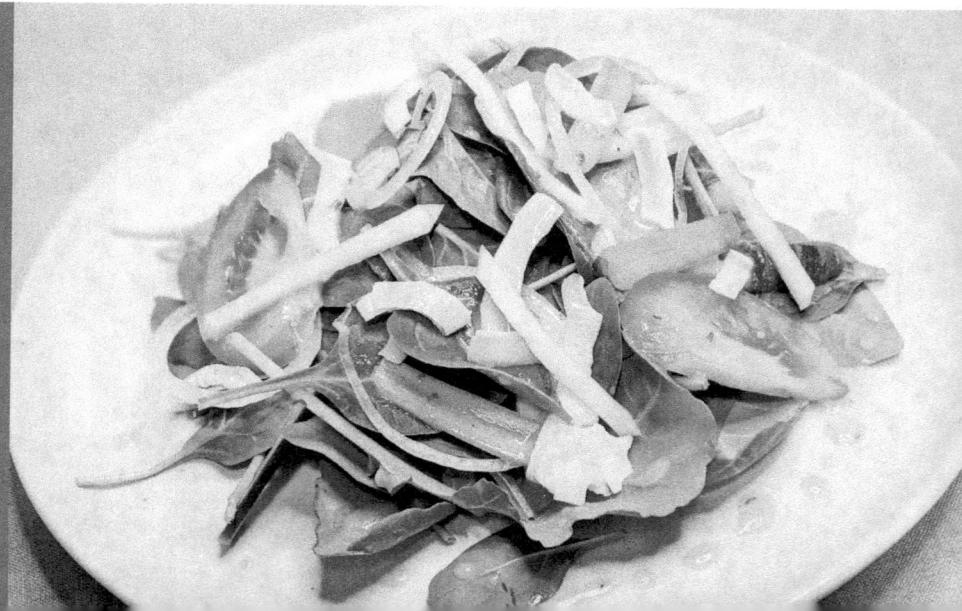

Vegetable Casserole

Prep Time: 10 minutes
Cook Time: 20minutes
Serves: 6
Difficulty Level: 1
Cost: $$

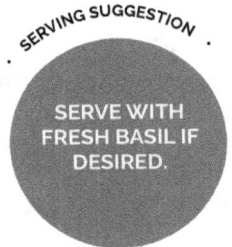

SERVING SUGGESTION

SERVE WITH FRESH BASIL IF DESIRED.

Ingredients:

- 1 zucchini, cut into quarters
- 1 red bell pepper, seeded and sliced
- 1 eggplant, cut into quarters
- 1 yellow onion, chopped
- 1 clove of garlic, chopped
- 3 tbsp olive oil
- 1 tbsp Italian seasoning
- Sea salt & pepper to taste
- Coconut oil for greasing

Directions:

1. Start by preheating the oven to 350 degrees F and grease a casserole dish with coconut oil.

2. Add all the vegetables to a large mixing bowl and drizzle with olive oil and season with the Italian seasoning, salt and pepper. Stir well.

3. Transfer the vegetables to the casserole dish and bake for 20 minutes or until the veggies are tender, tossing them halfway through.

4. Enjoy!

Nutritional Information:
Carbs: 9g
Fiber: 4g
Net Carbs: 5g
Protein: 2g
Fat: 8g
Calories: 106

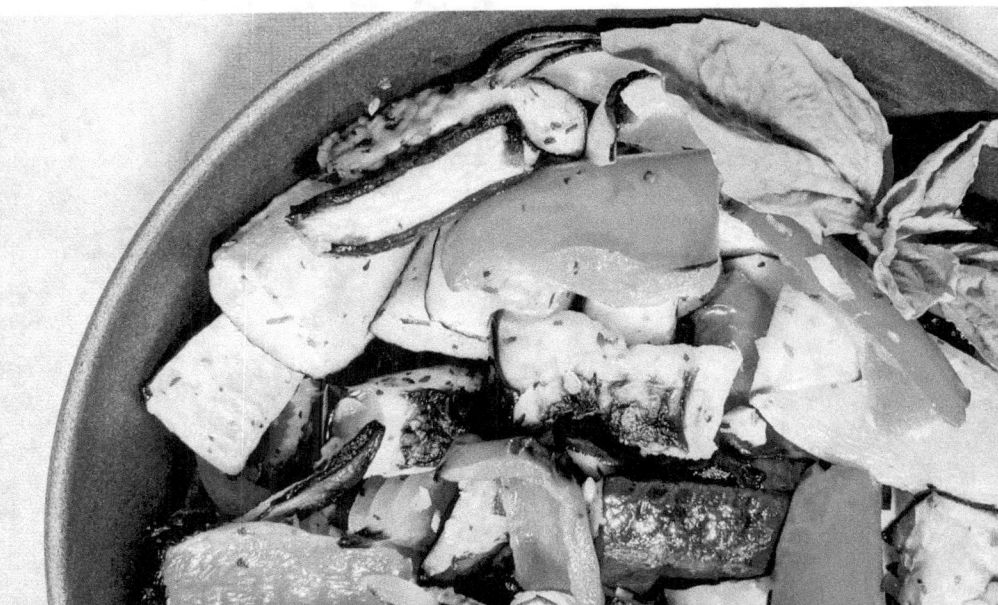

Balsamic Roasted Mushrooms

Prep Time: 10 minutes
Cook Time: 15-20 minutes
Serves: 4
Difficulty Level: 1
Cost: $$

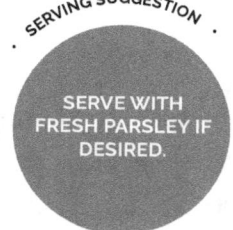

SERVING SUGGESTION

SERVE WITH FRESH PARSLEY IF DESIRED.

Ingredients:

- 2 cups mushrooms
- 2 tbsp olive oil
- 3 tbsp balsamic vinegar
- 1 tsp garlic powder
- Sea salt to taste

Directions:

1. Start by preheating the oven to 375 degrees F and line a baking sheet with parchment paper.

2. Add the mushrooms to a large mixing bowl with all the ingredients and toss well to combine, being sure to coat the mushrooms with the oil and seasoning.

3. Transfer to the baking sheet and bake for 15-20 minutes, tossing the mushrooms halfway through.

Nutritional Information:
Carbs: 2g
Fiber: 0g
Net Carbs: 2g
Protein: 1g
Fat: 7g
Calories: 72

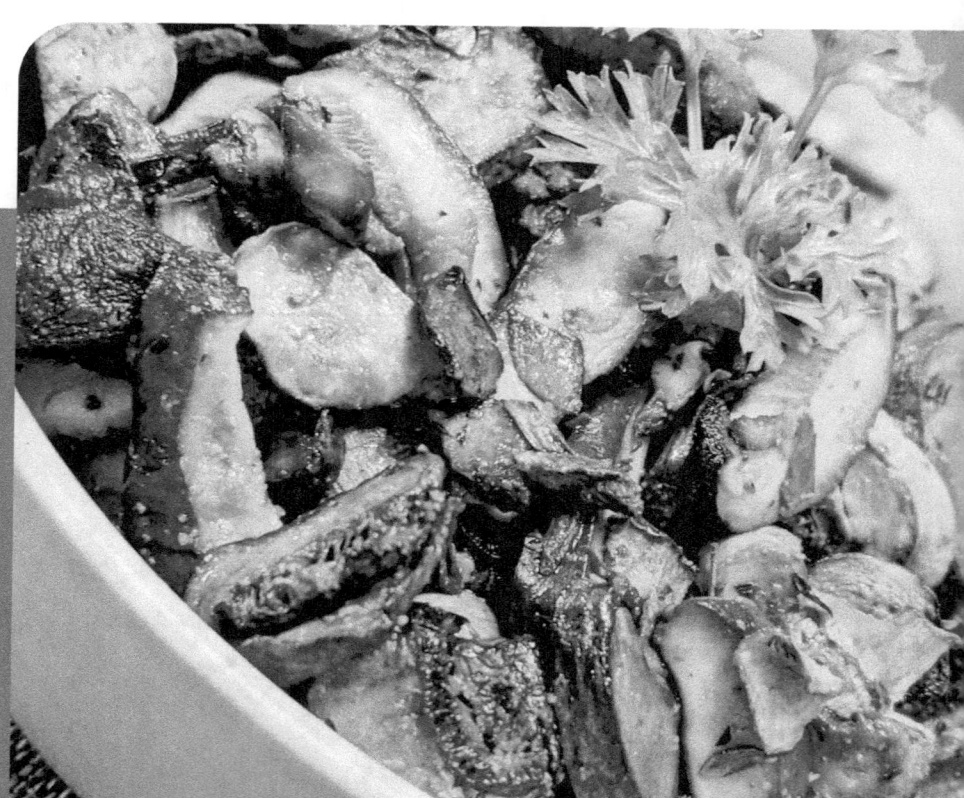

Dinner

Pepper & Onion Beef Soup

Prep Time: 10
Cook Time: 4-5 hours
Serves: 4
Difficulty Level: 1
Cost: $$

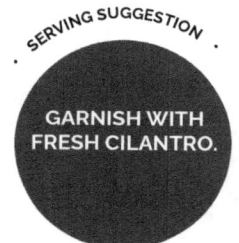

SERVING SUGGESTION

GARNISH WITH
FRESH CILANTRO.

Ingredients:

- 1 lb. lean beef chunks
- 4 cups reduced sodium beef broth
- 1 (14.5 oz.) can crushed tomatoes
- 1 red bell pepper, sliced
- 1 yellow onion, chopped
- 3 cloves garlic, chopped
- ½ cup carrots, sliced
- 1 zucchini, cut into rounds
- Salt & pepper to taste

Directions:

1. Add all of the ingredients to the base of the slow cooker.
2. Cook on low for 4–5 hours.

Nutritional Information:

Carbs: 9g

Fiber: 2g

Net Carbs: 7g

Protein: 17g

Fat: 13g

Calories: 222

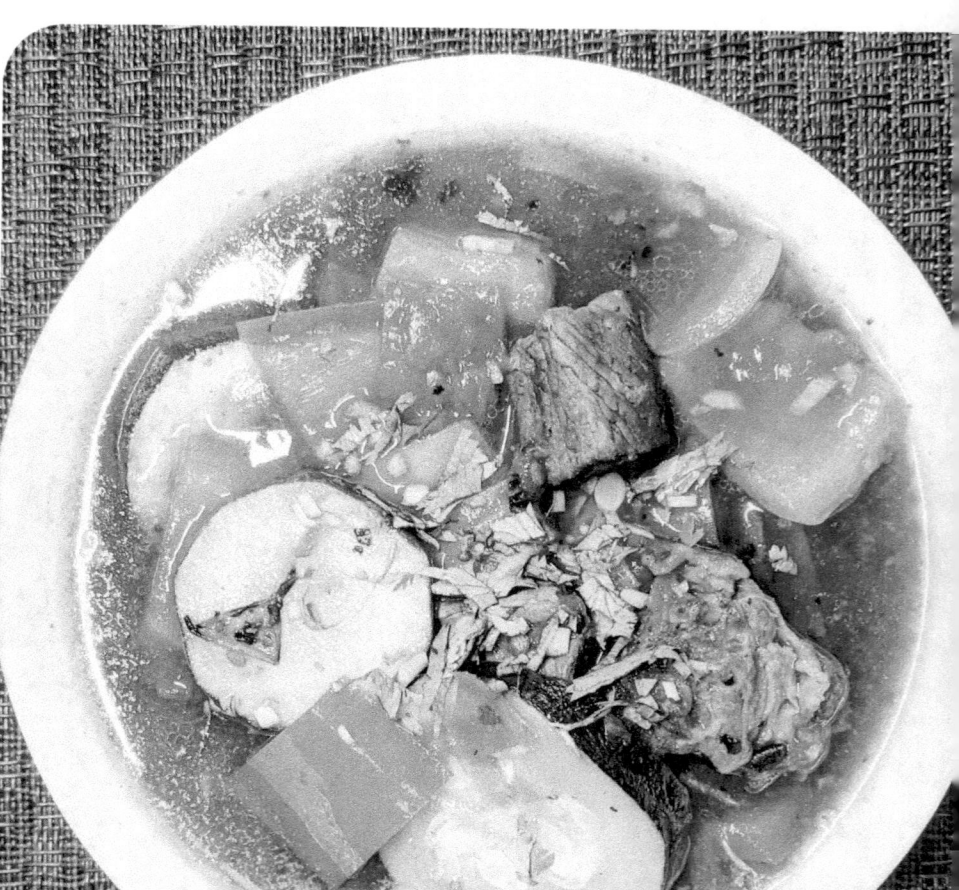

Garlicky Beef Stew

Prep Time: 10
Cook Time: 4-6 hours
Serves: 6
Difficulty Level: 1
Cost: $$

Ingredients:

- 2 lb. beef stew meat, cut into cubes
- ½ cup carrots, sliced
- ½ cup frozen peas
- 1 small white onion, chopped
- 2 green onions, thinly sliced
- 4 cloves garlic, chopped
- ½ tsp. sea salt
- ½ tsp. black pepper
- 1 ½ cups reduced sodium beef broth
- 1 tsp. Worcestershire sauce

Directions:

1. Start by adding the cubed beef to the base of the slow cooker and then top with the veggies.
2. Pour in the beef broth and cook on high for 4–6 hours.

SERVING SUGGESTION

SERVE WITH A SIDE OF STEAMED VEGETABLES SUCH AS BRUSSELS SPROUTS OR CAULIFLOWER.

Nutritional Information:
Carbs: 5g
Fiber: 1g
Net Carbs: 4g
Protein: 28g
Fat: 25g
Calories: 362

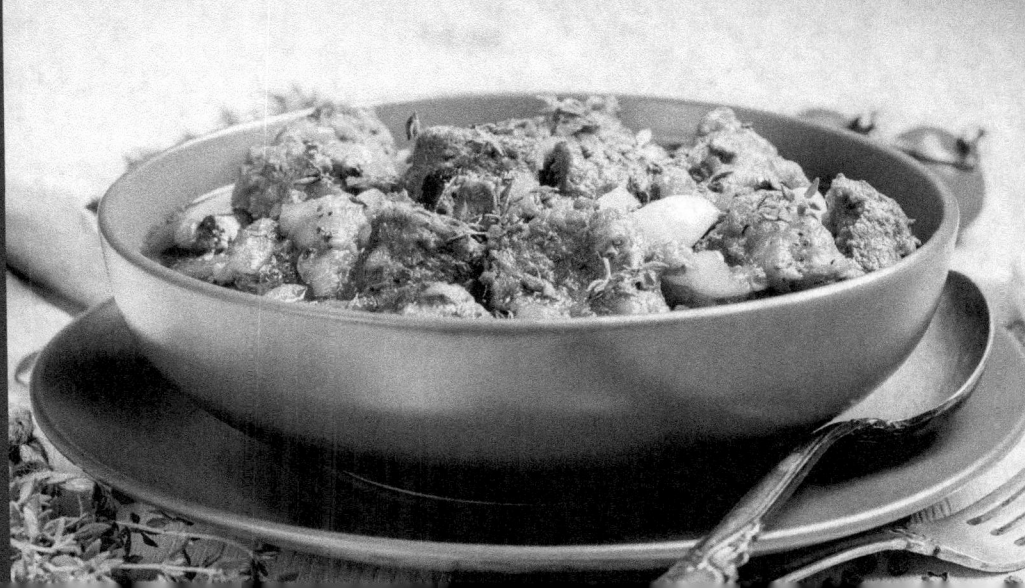

Lemon & Herb Whole Chicken

Prep Time: 10
Cook Time: 4-6 hours
Serves: 6
Difficulty Level: 1
Cost: $$

Ingredients:

- 1 whole (4 lb.) chicken
- 2 lemon wedges, sliced
- 4 cloves garlic, chopped
- 2 sprigs rosemary
- 1 tsp. dried thyme
- 1 tsp. onion powder
- ¼ tsp. black pepper
- 1 tsp. salt

Directions:

1. Start by mixing the thyme, onion powder, salt and pepper together in a small mixing bowl.

2. Rub the seasonings over the whole chicken and place the chicken into the slow cooker with the garlic, lemon wedges and rosemary sprigs.

3. Cook on low for 4–6 hours or until the juices run clear.

4. Remove the rosemary sprigs and lemon wedges before serving.

SERVING SUGGESTION

SQUEEZE EXTRA LEMON JUICE OVER THE CHICKEN BEFORE SERVING FOR AN EXTRA ZESTY FLAVOR AND SERVE WITH VEGGIES OF CHOICE.

Nutritional Information:
Carbs: 1g
Fiber: 0g
Net Carbs: 1g
Protein: 34g
Fat: 31g
Calories: 428

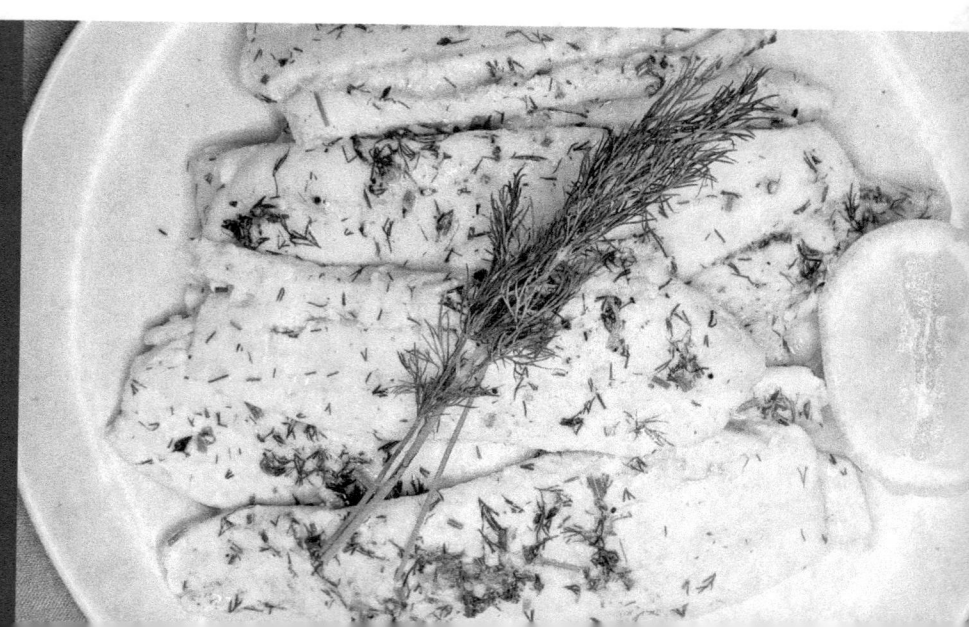

Peanut Curried Chicken

Prep Time: 10
Cook Time: 5 ½- 6 hours
Serves: 4
Difficulty Level: 1
Cost: $$

SERVING SUGGESTION

SERVE WITH STEAMED SNAP PEAS OR CAULIFLOWER AND GARNISH WITH FRESH BASIL IF DESIRED.

Ingredients:

- 4 boneless skinless chicken breasts, cubed
- 1 cup unsweetened full-fat coconut milk
- 1 tsp. curry powder
- 1 tsp. curry paste
- 2 Tbsp. peanut butter
- 2 Tbsp. coconut aminos
- 1 yellow onion, chopped
- 1 red bell pepper, sliced
- Spicy red chili pepper, chopped for garnish

Directions:

1. Start by whisking together the coconut milk, curry paste, curry powder, peanut butter and coconut aminos in the base of the slow cooker.

2. Next, add the remaining ingredients and cook on high for 5 ½–6 hours.

3. Garnish with spicy red pepper.

Nutritional Information:
Carbs: 9g
Fiber: 3g
Net Carbs: 6g
Protein: 31g
Fat: 22g
Calories: 348

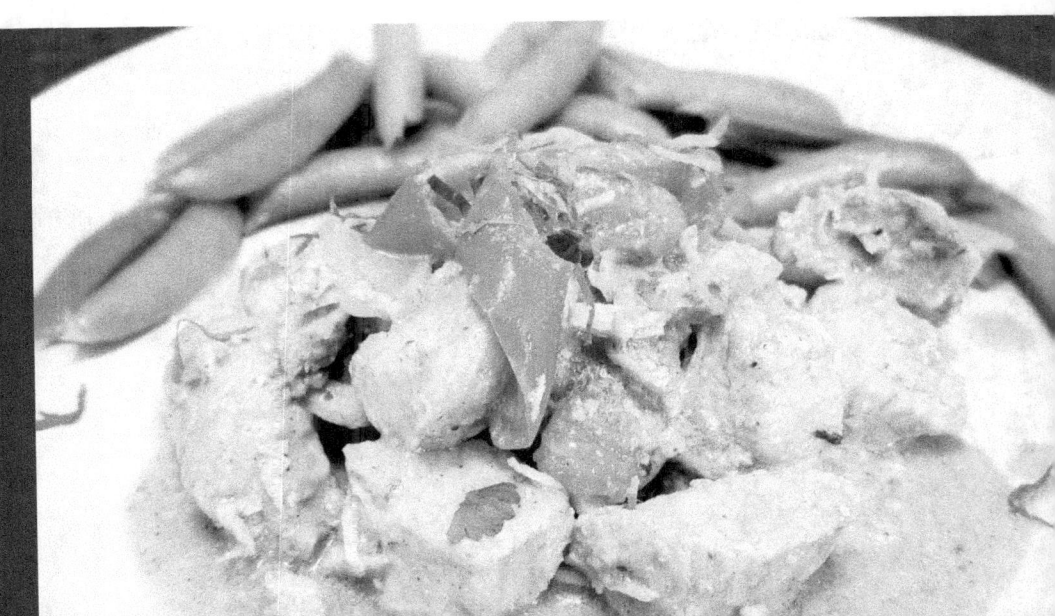

Minced Meat With Coconut Flour Tortillas

Prep Time: 15 minutes
Cook Time: 15 minutes
Serves: 4
Difficulty Level: 1
Cost: $$

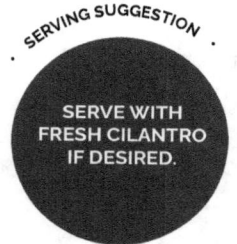

SERVING SUGGESTION

SERVE WITH
FRESH CILANTRO
IF DESIRED.

Nutritional Information:
Carbs: 10g
Fiber: 4g
Net Carbs: 6g
Protein: 22g
Fat: 29g
Calories: 378

Ingredients:

- Coconut Flour Tortilla Ingredients:
- ¼ cup coconut flour, sifted
- 2 eggs
- ½ cup unsweetened full-fat coconut milk
- 1 Tbsp. coconut oil for cooking
- Minced Meat Filling Ingredients:

- 1 lb. ground beef
- 4 Tbsp. tomato paste
- 1 tsp. cumin
- 1 tsp. paprika
- ½ tsp. black peppercorn, ground
- ½ tsp. salt
- 1 Tbsp. coconut oil

Directions:

1. Whisk all of the coconut tortilla ingredients together in a large mixing bowl. Let the batter sit for 5 minutes before cooking.

2. While the batter is sitting out, heat the coconut oil in a large skillet over low to medium heat. Pour a quarter of the mixture into the pan and cook for 1–2 minutes on each side until the sides begin to brown. Repeat this step with the remaining mixture.

3. Wipe a large skillet clean with paper towels and place over medium heat with the coconut oil from the minced meat filling ingredients.

4. Add the ground beef, tomato paste and seasonings into the skillet, and stir to combine.

5. Cook for 7–10 minutes or until the ground beef is cooked through.

6. Split into 4 servings, and serve with a coconut tortilla.

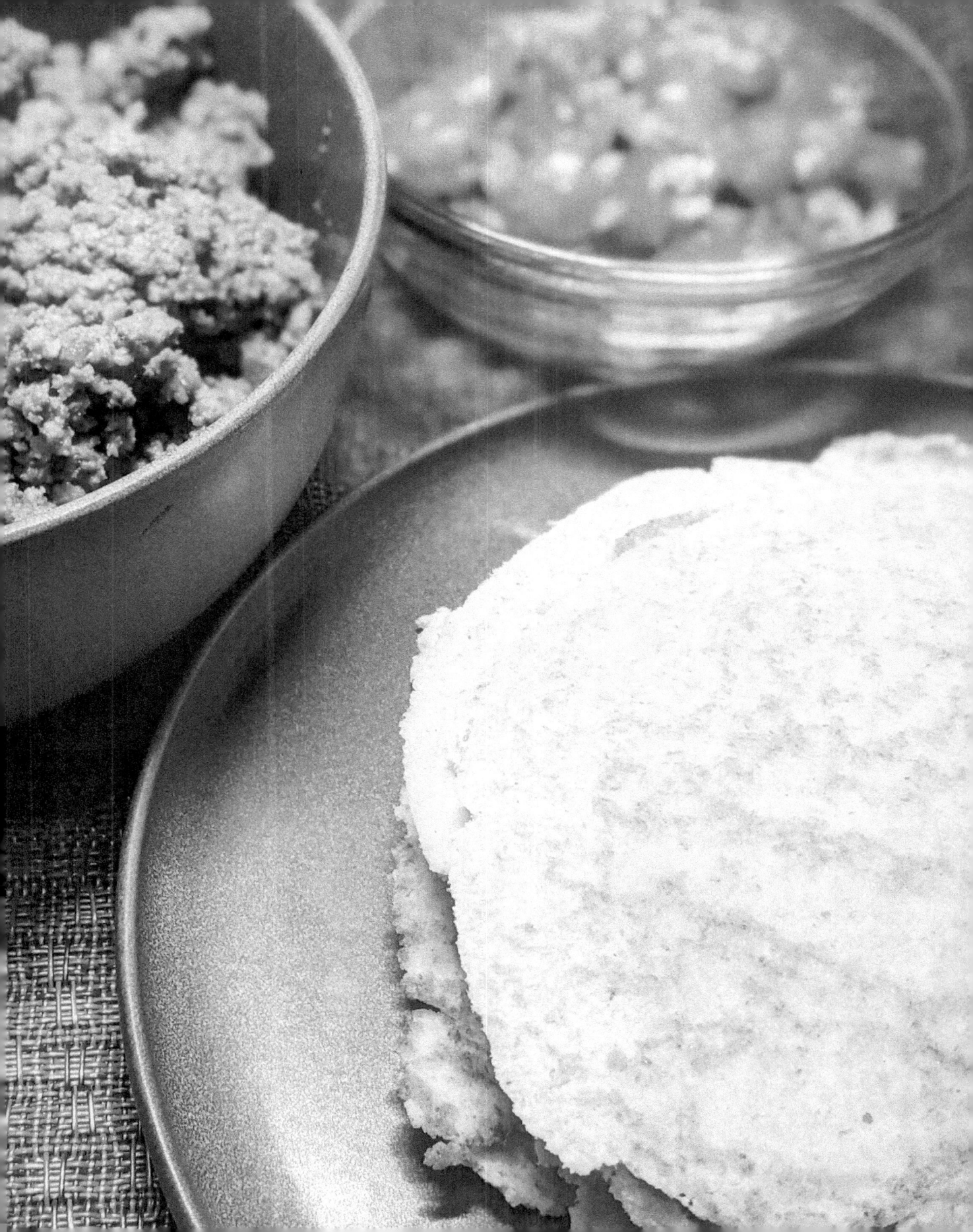

Herbed Green Bean Chicken Dish

Prep Time: 15 minutes
Cook Time: 25-30 minutes
Serves: 3
Difficulty Level: 1
Cost: $$

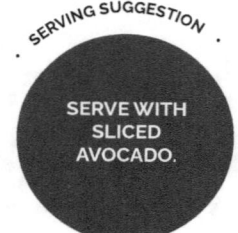

· SERVING SUGGESTION ·

SERVE WITH SLICED AVOCADO.

Ingredients:

- 2 whole chicken breasts
- 1 cup green beans, trimmed
- 8 cherry tomatoes, halved
- 2 Tbsp. olive oil
- 1 Tbsp. Italian seasoning
- 1 tsp. salt
- 1 tsp. black pepper

Directions:

1. Preheat a large skillet over medium heat with the olive oil.
2. Season the chicken with the Italian seasoning, salt and pepper.
3. Add the chicken to the skillet and cook for about 10 minutes each side or until cooked through.
4. Next, add the green beans and tomatoes and cook for another 5–7 minutes.
5. Enjoy right away.

Nutritional Information:
Carbs: 6g
Fiber: 2g
Net Carbs: 4g
Protein: 19g
Fat: 11g
Calories: 196

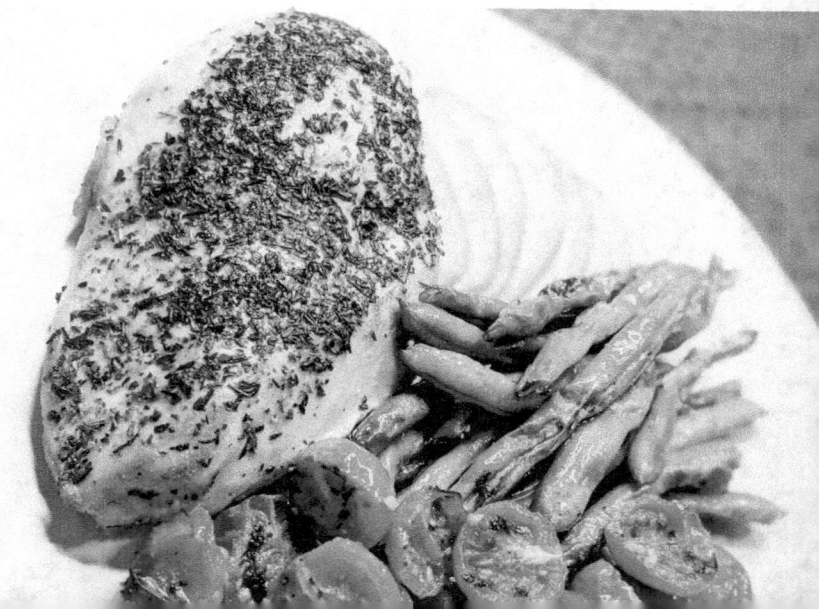

Garlic & Thyme Lamb Chops

Prep Time: 15 minutes
Cook Time: 20-25 minutes
Serves: 6
Difficulty Level: 1
Cost: $$

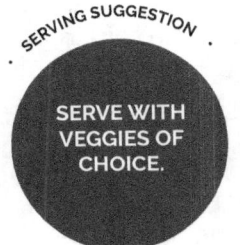

SERVING SUGGESTION

SERVE WITH VEGGIES OF CHOICE.

Ingredients:

- 6 (4 oz.) lamb chops
- 4 cloves garlic, whole
- 3 Tbsp. olive oil
- 1 tsp. ground thyme
- 2 sprigs of thyme
- 1 tsp. salt
- 1 tsp. black pepper

Directions:

1. Preheat a large skillet over medium heat with the olive oil.
2. Season the lamb chops with the salt, pepper and thyme.
3. Add the lamb chops to the pan with the thyme sprigs and garlic.
4. Cook about 3–4 minutes on each side.
5. Enjoy right away.

Nutritional Information:
Carbs: 1g
Fiber: 0g
Net Carbs: 1g
Protein: 14g
Fat: 21g
Calories: 252

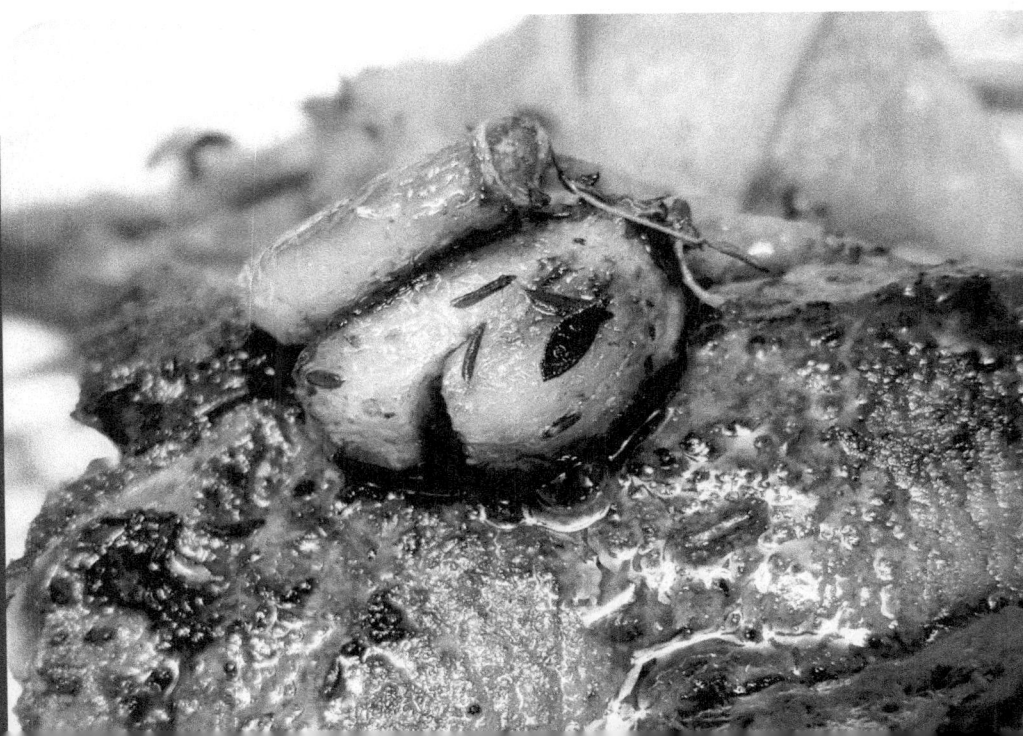

Sesame Fried Tofu

Prep Time: 15 minutes
Cook Time: 15 minutes
Serves: 4
Difficulty Level: 1
Cost: $$

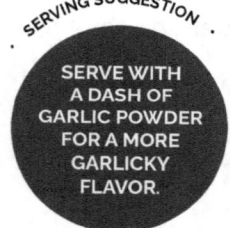

SERVING SUGGESTION

SERVE WITH
A DASH OF
GARLIC POWDER
FOR A MORE
GARLICKY
FLAVOR.

Ingredients:

- 1 (14 oz.) package extra firm tofu
- 6 cups fresh spinach
- 3 cloves garlic, chopped
- ¼ cup coconut aminos
- 2 tsp. sesame oil
- 2 Tbsp. sesame seeds
- 1 Tbsp. coconut oil

Directions:

1. Remove the tofu block from the container and press (see cooking tips on how to press tofu). Next, cut the tofu into cubes.

2. Add the coconut aminos and sesame oil to a mixing bowl and add the tofu cubes. Allow the tofu to absorb the marinade for 5–10 minutes.

3. Next, preheat a large skillet over medium heat with the coconut oil. Add the tofu cubes and sauté for 7–8 minutes or until golden brown.

4. Add the garlic and spinach. Sauté for another 3–5 minutes or until the spinach is wilted.

5. Place into a large serving bowl and top with sesame seeds.

6. Split into four servings and enjoy

Nutritional Information:
Carbs: 6g
Fiber: 2g
Net Carbs: 4g
Protein: 13g
Fat: 14g
Calories: 188

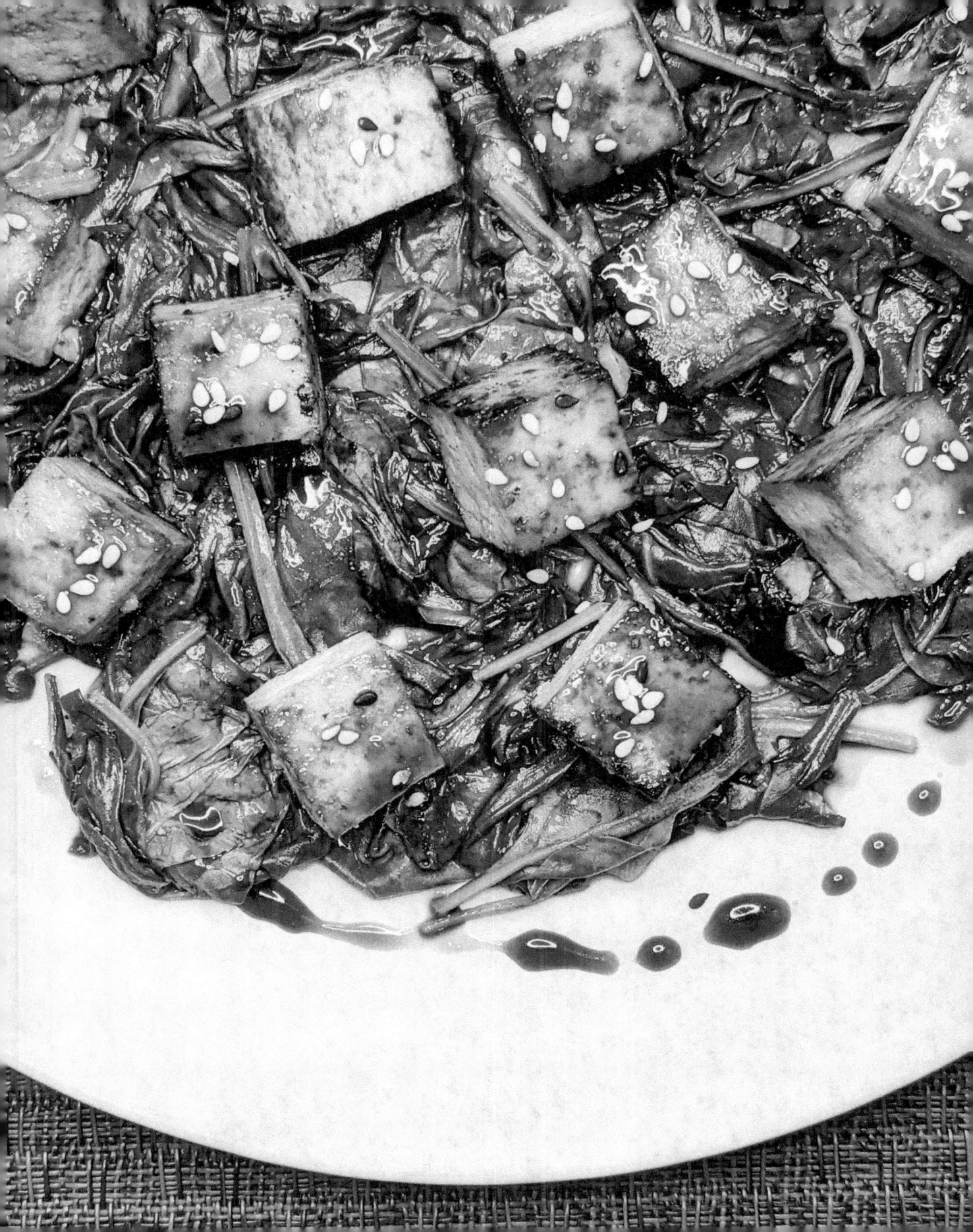

Wild Dill Salmon

Prep Time: 10 minutes
Cook Time: 2 hours
Serves: 4
Difficulty Level: 1
Cost: $$$

SERVING SUGGESTION

SERVE WITH A SALAD OR WITH STEAMED BROCCOLI OR GREEN BEANS. ADD AN EXTRA SQUEEZE OF FRESH LEMON JUICE IF DESIRED.

Ingredients:

- 2 lbs. skin-on wild caught salmon
- 2 cups water
- 1 cup reduced sodium vegetable broth
- 1 lemon, thinly sliced
- 1 onion, finely chopped
- 3 sprigs dill
- Salt & pepper to taste

Directions:

1. Simply place all of the ingredients into a slow cooker, adding the salmon to the base of the slow cooker and then adding the remaining ingredients.
2. Cook for 2 hours on high or until the fish begins to flake.

Nutritional Information:

Carbs: 3g

Fiber: 1g

Net Carbs: 2g

Protein: 50g

Fat: 13g

Calories: 341

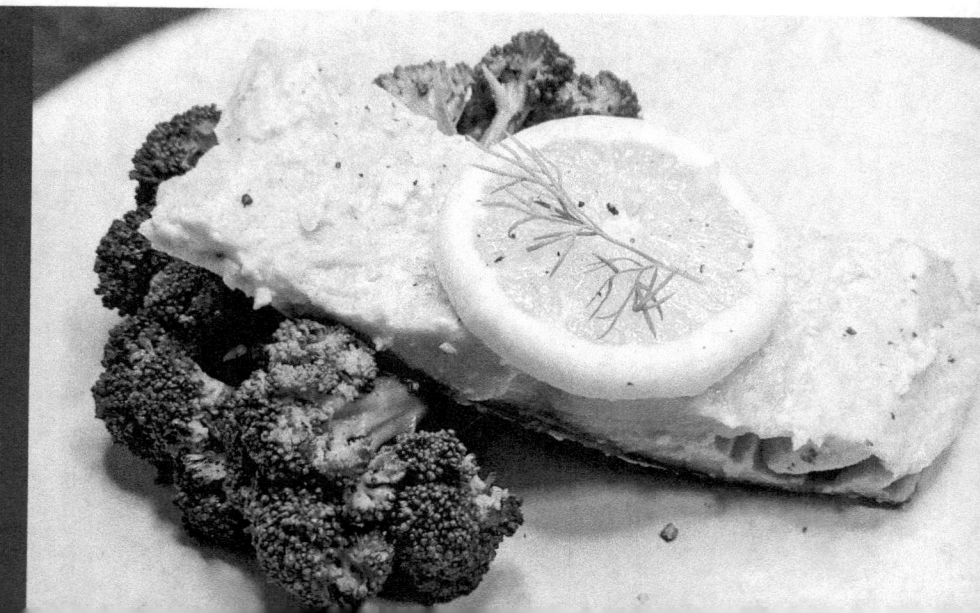

Balsamic Meatloaf

Prep Time: 10 minutes
Cook Time: 60 minutes
Serves: 6
Difficulty Level: 2
Cost: $$

SERVING SUGGESTION

SERVE WITH BROCCOLI OR VEGETABLE OF CHOICE!

Ingredients:

- 1 lb. ground beef
- 1 yellow onion, finely chopped
- 2 cloves garlic, chopped
- 2 Tbsp. tomato paste
- ¼ cup balsamic vinegar (gluten free)
- 1 Tbsp. Italian seasoning
- 1 tsp. salt
- ½ tsp. black pepper
- Coconut oil for greasing

Directions:

1. Start by preheating the oven to 350°F and greasing a 9 x 5 loaf pan with coconut oil.

2. Add all of the ingredients to a large mixing bowl and mix well.

3. Add the mixture to the greased loaf pan and bake for 55-60 minutes or until the meatloaf is cooked all the way through.

4. Cool for 10 minutes before slicing.

Nutritional Information:
Carbs: 4g
Fiber: 1g
Net Carbs: 3g
Protein: 24g
Fat: 6g
Calories: 163

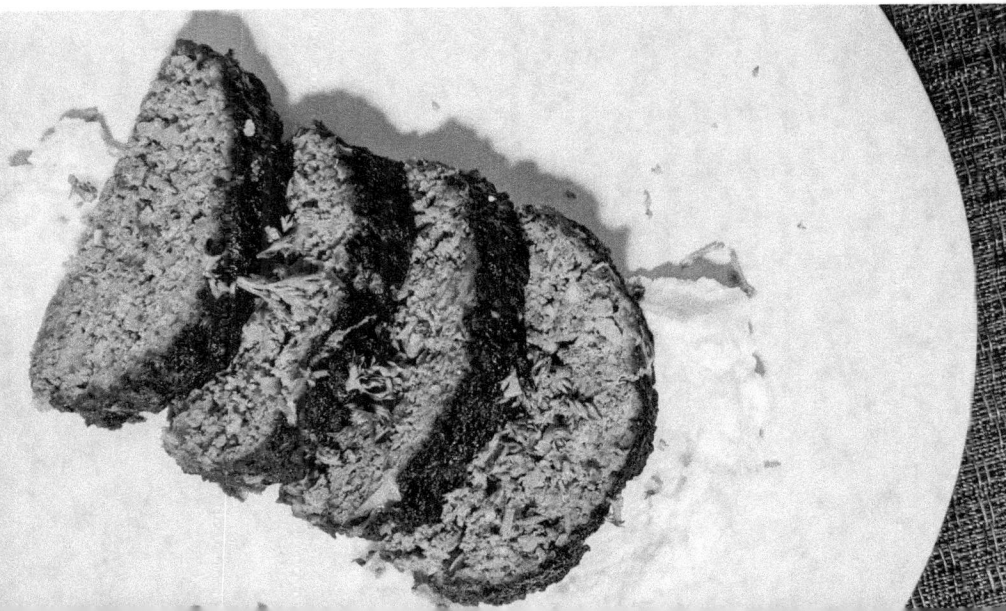

Herb Fried Chicken

Prep Time: 15 minutes
Cook Time: 20-25 minutes
Serves: 4
Difficulty Level: 2
Cost: $

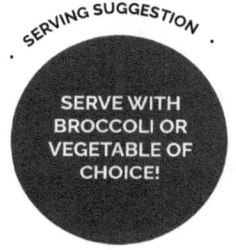

SERVING SUGGESTION

SERVE WITH BROCCOLI OR VEGETABLE OF CHOICE!

Ingredients:

- 4 boneless skinless chicken breasts
- 1 egg
- ½ cup almond flour
- ½ tsp. onion powder
- 1 tsp. garlic powder
- 1 Tbsp. Italian seasoning
- ½ tsp. paprika
- 1 tsp. salt
- Coconut oil for greasing

Directions:

1. Start by preheating the oven to 350°F and greasing a baking dish with coconut oil.

2. Add the egg to a small bowl and then add the almond flour with the seasoning to another bowl.

3. Dip the chicken breasts into the egg mixture, covering both sides, and then dip into the almond flour mixture, again covering both sides.

4. Add the chicken breasts to the baking dish and bake for 20-25 minutes or until the chicken is no longer pink in the middle. Flip the chicken halfway through.

Nutritional Information:
Carbs: 2g
Fiber: 1g
Net Carbs: 1g
Protein: 45g
Fat: 15g
Calories: 328

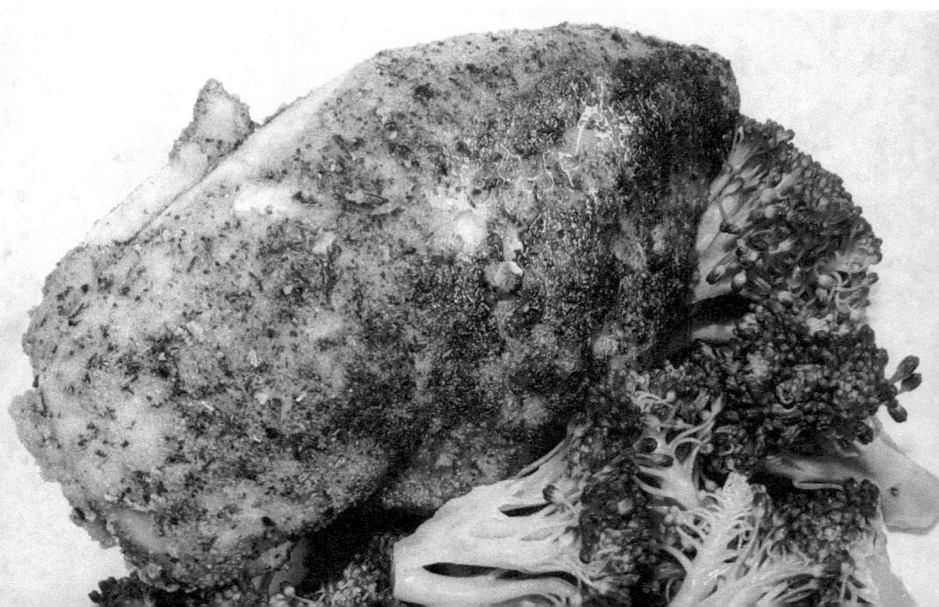

Caribbean Chicken

Prep Time: 10 minutes
Cook Time: 20 minutes
Serves: 4
Difficulty Level: 2
Cost: $$

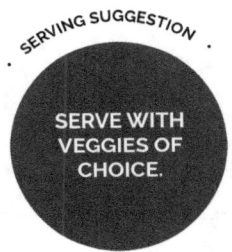

SERVING SUGGESTION

SERVE WITH VEGGIES OF CHOICE.

Ingredients:

- 4 chicken breasts (with bone and skin)
- 1 red onion, peeled and chopped
- 4 Tbsp. melted coconut oil
- 1 Tbsp. soy sauce
- 1 Tbsp. lime zest
- 2 tsp. ground ginger
- 1 Tbsp. jalapeño pepper, seeded and chopped
- Juice of 1 lime
- 1 lime, cut into wedges, for serving (optional)

Directions:

1. Puree all of the ingredients in a food processor except for the chicken breasts.

2. Transfer the marinade to a bowl and add the chicken breasts. Let this marinate for at least 2 hours in the refrigerator before cooking.

3. After the chicken has marinated, heat up your grill, and grill each side of the chicken for about 10 minutes or until the chicken is thoroughly cooked.

4. Serve with a fresh lime wedge, if desired.

Nutritional Information:
Carbs: 3g
Fiber: 0g
Net Carbs: 3g
Protein: 27g
Fat: 17g
Calories: 268

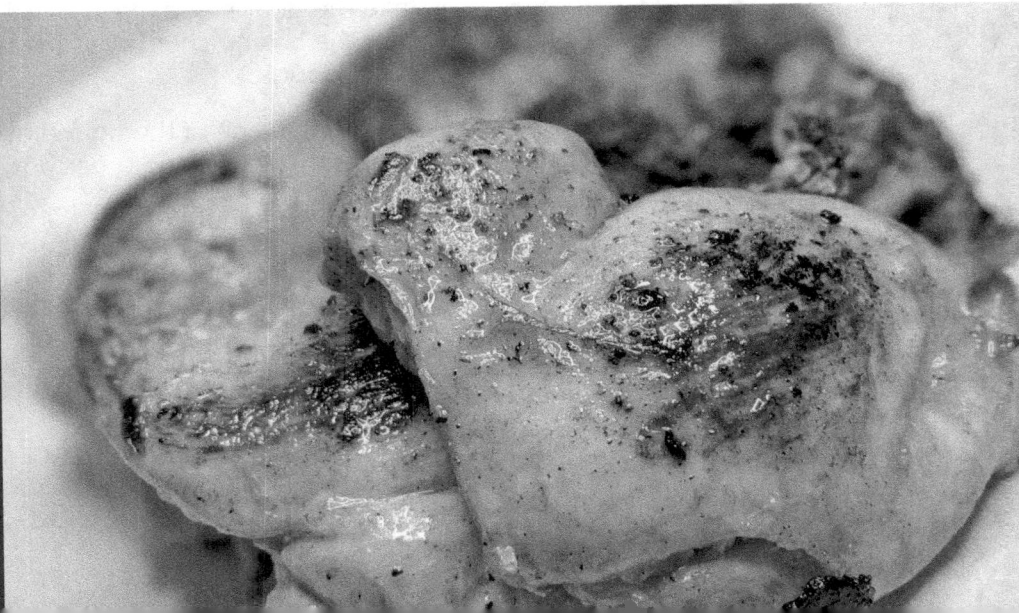

Jamaican Patties

Prep Time: 20 minutes
Cook Time: 30 minutes
Serves: 2
Difficulty Level: 2
Cost: $$

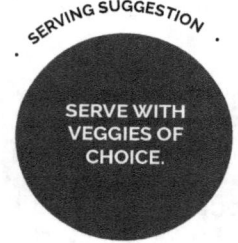

SERVING SUGGESTION

SERVE WITH VEGGIES OF CHOICE.

Nutritional Information:

Carbs: 13g

Fiber: 2g

Net Carbs: 11g

Protein: 14g

Fat: 23g

Calories: 307

Ingredients:

- 2 eggs
- ½ cup coconut milk
- 2 Tbsp. coconut oil
- ½ cup coconut flour
- ½ tsp. baking powder
- 1 tsp. turmeric
- ½ pound ground beef
- ½ onion, peeled and chopped
- 1 pinch cumin
- 1 pinch salt and ground black pepper
- 1 jalapeño pepper, seeded and chopped

Directions:

1. Whisk the milk and eggs until well combined.

2. Add the coconut oil and coconut fl our and whisk. Add the turmeric, salt, and black pepper. Mix until smooth.

3. Sauté the onion in a pan with the ground beef, cumin, and chopped jalapeño pepper. Cook until the meat is no longer pink.

4. Preheat your oven to 350 degrees, and line a baking sheet with parchment paper.

5. Take the dough and make 4 balls, and roll the dough flat onto the baking sheet. Add the beef mixture on two pieces of the dough.

6. Place one piece of the dough over another to create 2 large Jamaican patties, and press down to seal the edges.

7. Bake for 30 minutes.

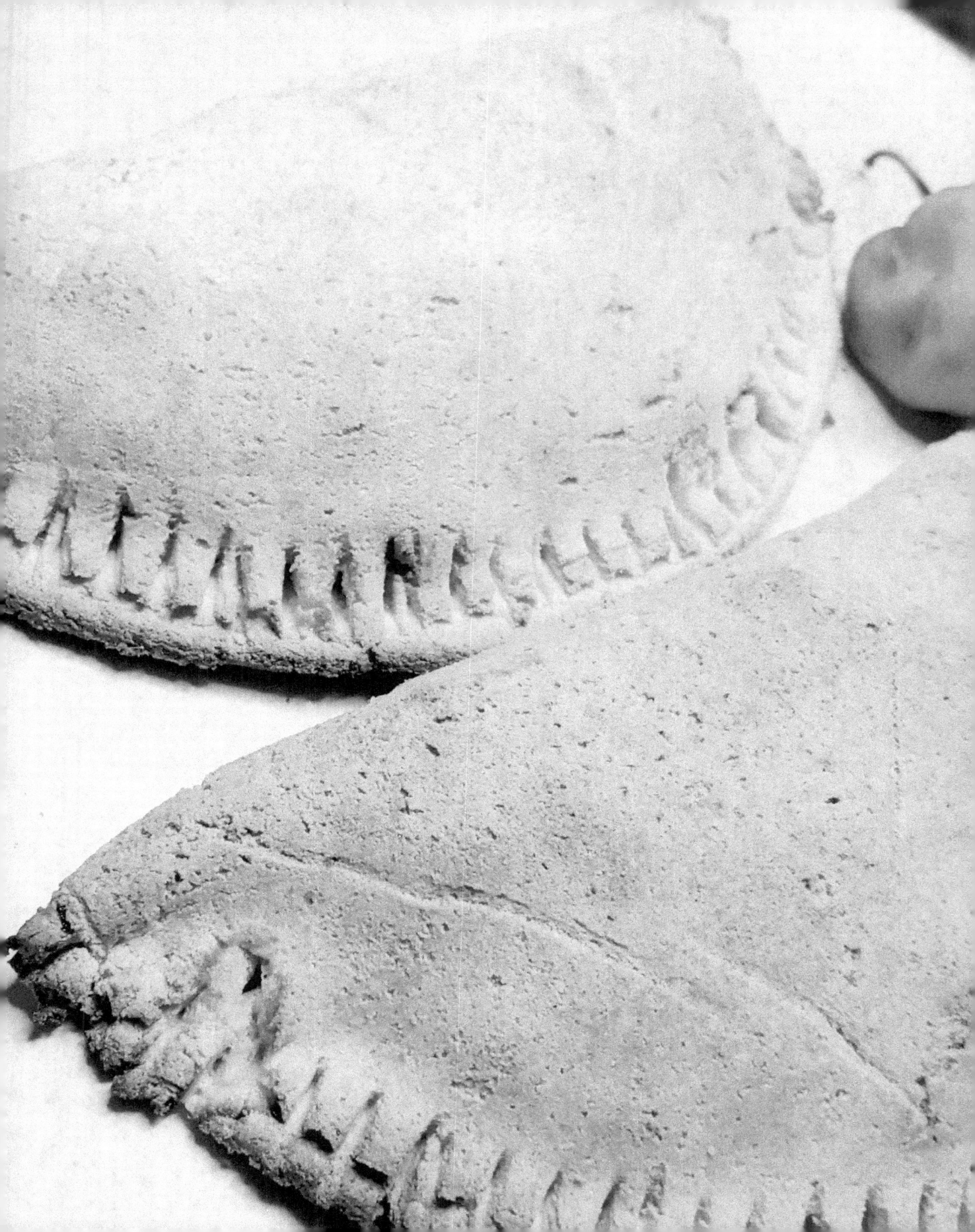

Blackened Salmon

Prep Time: 20 minutes
Cook Time: 25 minutes
Serves: 2
Difficulty Level: 2
Cost: $$$

SERVING SUGGESTION

SERVE WITH STEAMED BROCCOLI IF DESIRED.

Ingredients:

- 2 salmon fillets
- 1 avocado
- 1 Tbsp. mayonnaise
- 1 Tbsp. blackening spice
- 1 cup lettuce
- 1 pinch sea salt

Directions:

1. Mash the avocado and add the mayonnaise, mixing until combined.
2. Preheat the grill.
3. While the grill is heating up, rub the seasonings on both sides of the salmon fi llets, and place them on the grill. Grill for about 5 minutes per side or until cooked.
4. Serve over lettuce and top with the avocado sauce.

Nutritional Information:
Carbs: 4g
Fiber: 3g
Net Carbs: 1g
Protein: 51g
Fat: 38g
Calories: 568

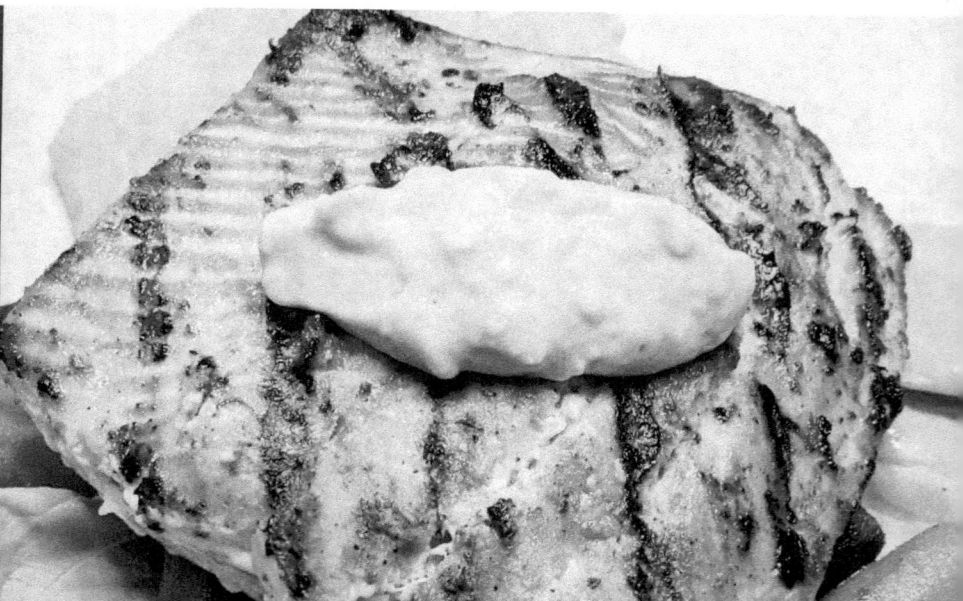

Thai Chicken Soup

Prep Time: 10 minutes
Cook Time: 30 minutes
Serves: 4
Difficulty Level: 2
Cost: $$

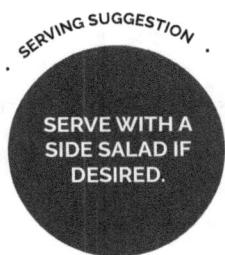

SERVING SUGGESTION

SERVE WITH A SIDE SALAD IF DESIRED.

Ingredients:

- 2 chicken breasts, thinly sliced
- 1 (15-ounce) can coconut milk
- 1 onion, peeled and chopped
- 3 garlic cloves, peeled and minced
- 6 cups chicken broth
- 2 Tbsp. green curry paste
- 1 Tbsp. fish sauce
- 2 carrots, peeled and cut into crescents
- 1 zucchini, cut into rounds
- Pinch of sea salt
- 1 Tbsp. olive oil

Directions:

1. Heat a large stockpot over medium heat and add the olive oil. Start to sauté the onion for 2 to 4 minutes. Add the garlic and sauté for another minute.

2. Add the remaining ingredients and bring to a boil.

3. Simmer for 20 to 25 minutes or until the chicken is cooked through and the vegetables are tender.

4. Serve right away.

Nutritional Information:
Carbs: 17g
Fiber: 5g
Net Carbs: 12g
Protein: 19g
Fat: 35g
Calories: 430

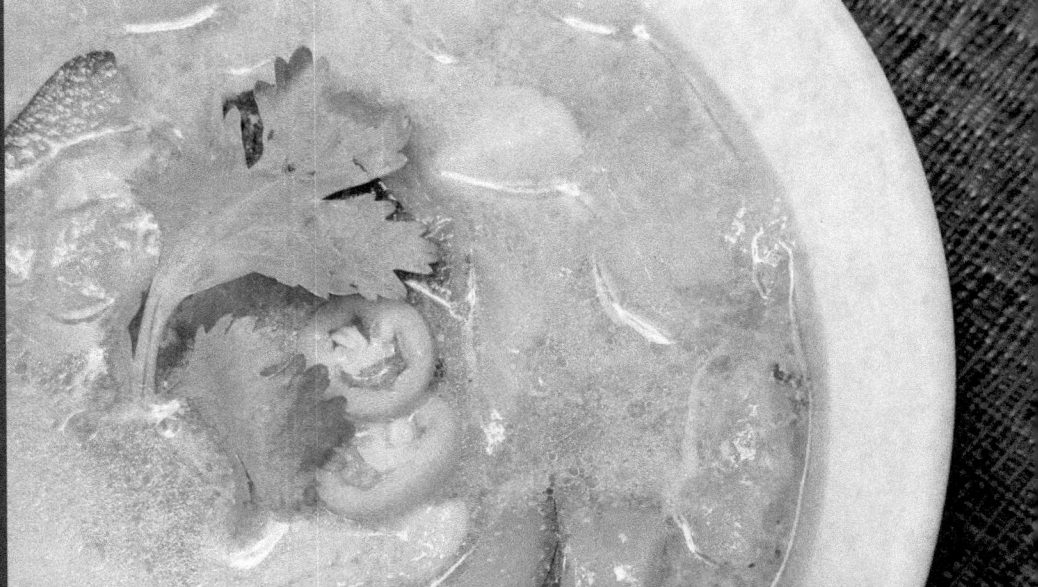

General Tso's Chicken

Prep Time: 15 minutes
Cook Time: 10 minutes
Serves: 5
Difficulty Level: 2
Cost: $$

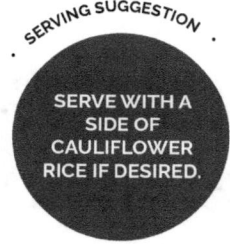

SERVING SUGGESTION

SERVE WITH A SIDE OF CAULIFLOWER RICE IF DESIRED.

Ingredients:

- 6 boneless and skinless chicken breasts, cubed
- ½ cup almond flour
- 1 egg
- 3 Tbsp. coconut oil
- 2 Tbsp. chicken broth
- 2 Tbsp. rice vinegar
- 2 Tbsp. soy sauce
- ¼ tsp. sesame oil
- ½ tsp. onion powder
- 1 tsp. red pepper flakes
- 1 pinch ground ginger
- Green onions, for garnish

Directions:

1. In a large bowl, combine the rice vinegar, soy sauce, sesame oil, chicken broth, red pepper flakes, onion powder, and ginger and set aside.

2. In a separate bowl, whisk the egg and set aside.

3. In another bowl, add the almond fl our.

4. Take the chicken cubes, dip them into the almond fl our and cover on both sides. Dip into the egg mixture to cover. Add to the dressing mixture to thoroughly cover both sides.

5. In a large sauté pan, heat the oil over medium heat, then add the leftover soy sauce mixture and a pinch of almond fl our to thicken up the sauce a bit.

6. Add the chicken cubes and sauté for about 7 minutes on each side or until well browned and cooked through.

7. Serve with green onions, if desired.

Nutritional Information:
Carbs: 3g
Fiber: 2g
Net Carbs: 1g
Protein: 36g
Fat: 22g
Calories: 355

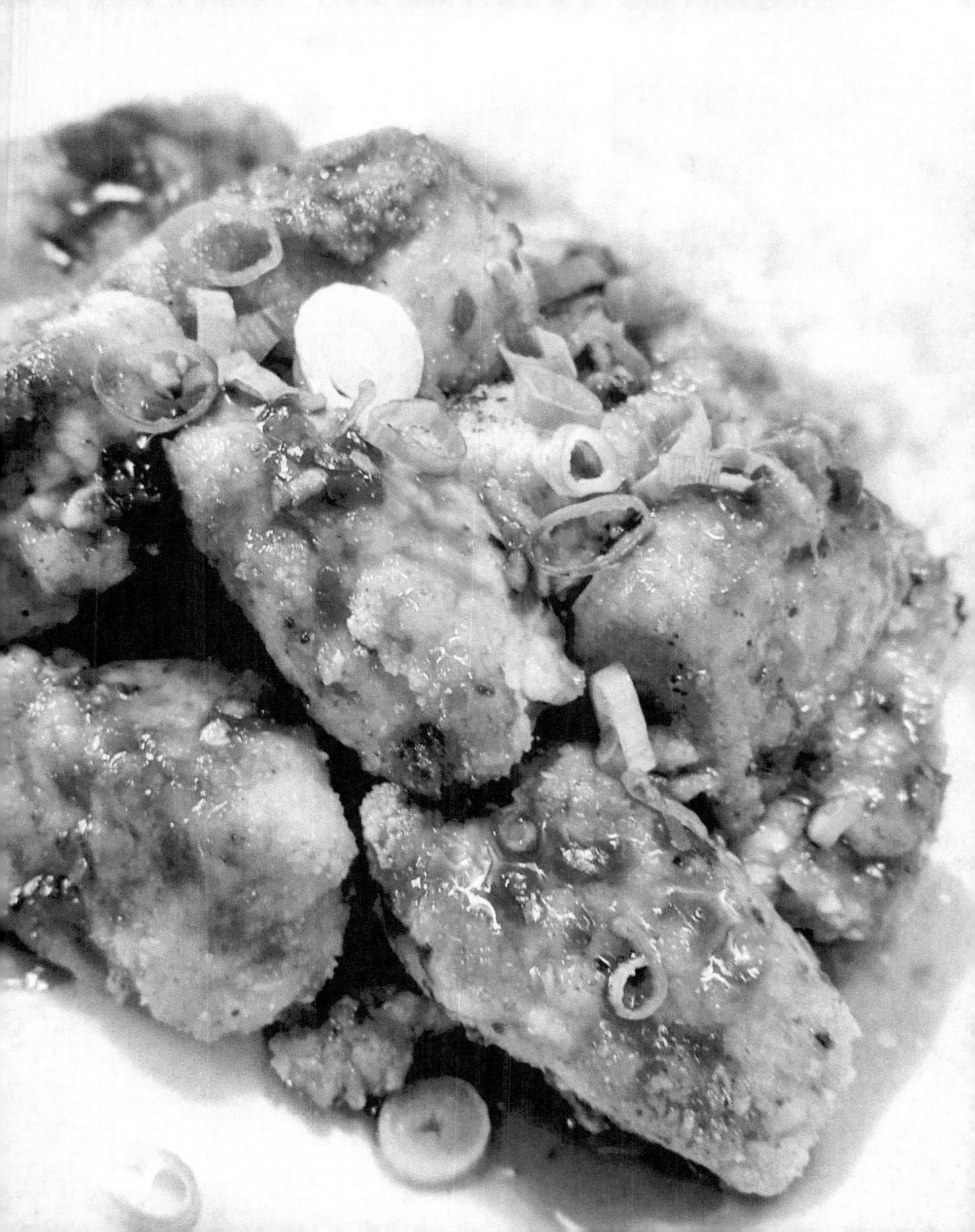

Beef & Broccoli

Prep Time: 15 minutes
Cook Time: 10 minutes
Serves: 4
Difficulty Level: 2
Cost: $$

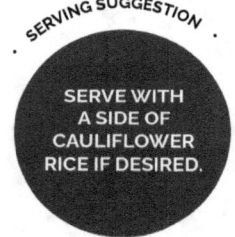

SERVING SUGGESTION

SERVE WITH
A SIDE OF
CAULIFLOWER
RICE IF DESIRED.

Nutritional Information:

Carbs: 12g

Fiber: 1g

Net Carbs: 11g

Protein: 30g

Fat: 15g

Calories: 296

Ingredients:

- ½ cup low-sodium soy sauce
- ¼ cup cornstarch
- ½ Tbsp. freshly grated ginger
- 1 Tbsp. garlic powder
- 1 pound flank steak, sliced thinly
- 2 Tbsp. peanut oil
- 2 cups broccoli florets
- 2 Tbsp. fish sauce
- ¼ cup shredded cabbage, for garnish

Directions:

1. Put the sliced beef in a mixing bowl and set aside.

2. In a separate bowl, add the soy sauce, fish sauce, cornstarch, ginger, and garlic. Pour ½ of this mixture over the beef.

3. Heat a large skillet over medium heat with 1 tablespoon of peanut oil and add the broccoli. Sauté for 2 minutes and then place on a serving plate.

4. In the same skillet, pour the rest of the remaining 1 tablespoon of peanut oil and add the beef. Cook for about 1 minute on each side until brown.

5. Add the remaining sauce mixture, and cook on high heat until the sauce starts to thicken.

6. Add the broccoli back to the skillet and stir to combine.

7. Serve on 4 different serving plates, and top with shredded cabbage, if desired.

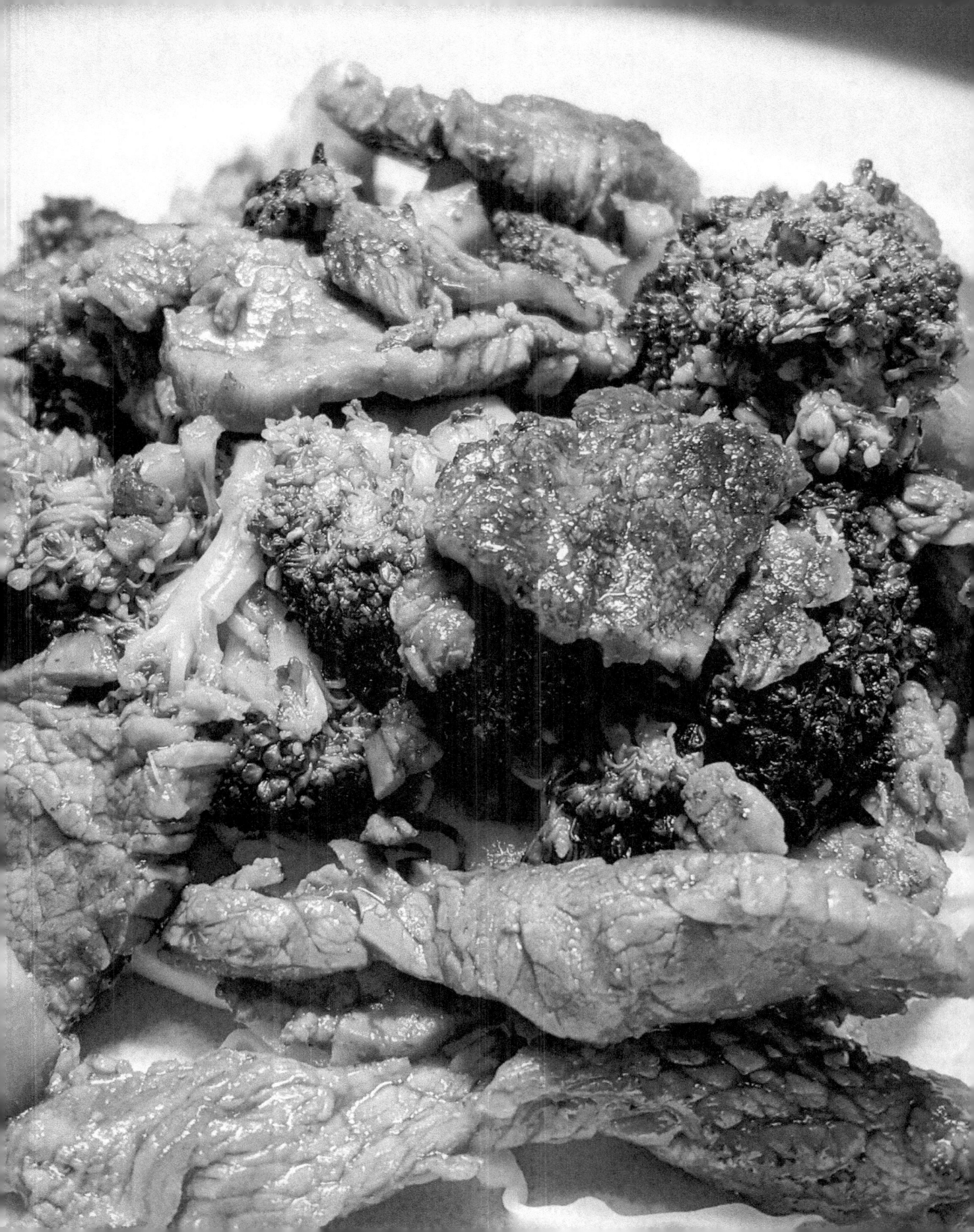

Garlic Shrimp

Prep Time: 10 minutes
Cook Time: 10 minutes
Serves: 3
Difficulty Level: 2
Cost: $$

SERVING SUGGESTION

SERVE WITH STEAMED BROCCOLI AND AVOCADO FOR ADDED HEALTHY FAT IF DESIRED.

Ingredients:

- 1 pound peeled and deveined shrimp, tails left on
- 2 Tbsp. fish sauce
- 1 Tbsp. soy sauce
- 1 tsp. sesame oil
- 1 Tbsp. cornstarch
- 4 garlic cloves, peeled and chopped
- 2 green onions, finely chopped, for garnish
- 1 Tbsp. peanut oil, for cooking

Directions:

1. Whisk together the fish sauce, soy sauce, sesame oil, garlic, and cornstarch in a mixing bowl until smooth.

2. Preheat a large skillet over medium heat with the peanut oil. Once heated, add the shrimp and sauté for 3 to 5 minutes, flipping the shrimp halfway through.

3. Pour in the sauce mixture and simmer for 5 minutes or until the sauce starts to thicken up.

4. Serve topped with freshly chopped green onions.

Nutritional Information:
Carbs: 7g
Fiber: 0g
Net Carbs: 7g
Protein: 22g
Fat: 8g
Calories: 185

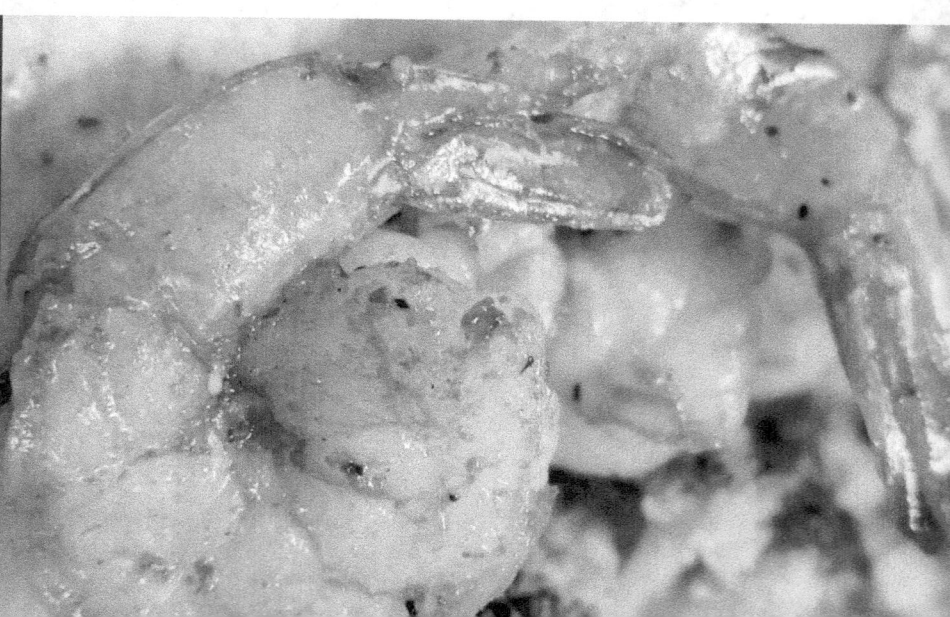

Irish Lamb Stew

Prep Time: 20 minutes

Cook Time: 30 minutes

Serves: 6

Difficulty Level: 2

Cost: $$

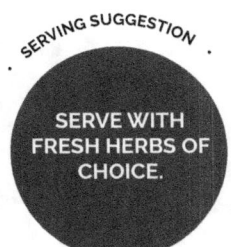

SERVING SUGGESTION

SERVE WITH FRESH HERBS OF CHOICE.

Ingredients:

- 8 small lamb chops
- 1 onion, peeled and chopped
- 1 tsp. black peppercorns
- 1 tsp. fresh rosemary
- 1 tsp. fresh thyme
- 1 leek, chopped (white part only)
- 1 cup button mushrooms
- 4 garlic cloves, peeled and minced
- 4 cups vegetable broth
- 1 cup chopped carrots
- 1 Tbsp. coconut oil

Directions:

1. Start by heating a large skillet over medium heat with the coconut oil and brown the lamb chops. Add the leek and garlic and cook for another 3 minutes.

2. Add all of the ingredients including the lamb, leek, and garlic to a large stockpot and simmer for 25 minutes.

Nutritional Information:

Carbs: 8g

Fiber: 1g

Net Carbs: 7g

Protein: 20g

Fat: 22g

Calories: 309

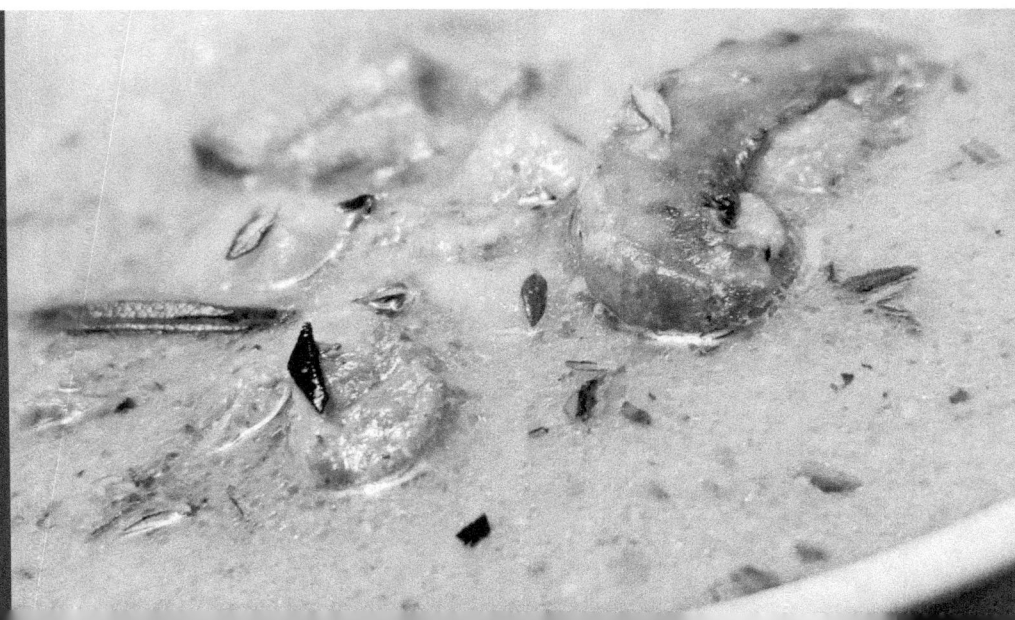

Desserts

Raspberry Avocado Ice Cream

Prep Time: 5 minutes
Cook Time: 0 minutes
Serves: 2
Difficulty Level: 1
Cost: $$

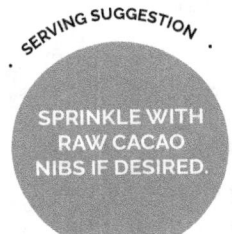

SERVING SUGGESTION

SPRINKLE WITH RAW CACAO NIBS IF DESIRED.

Ingredients:

- 1 cup frozen strawberries
- 1 avocado, pitted and cubed
- ¼ cup full-fat unsweetened coconut milk
- 1 tsp pure vanilla extract
- Zero carb sweetener of choice

Directions:

1. Add all ingredients to a blender or food processor and blend until creamy.
2. Serve right away.

Nutritional Information:
Carbs: 16g
Fiber: 9g
Net Carbs: 7g
Protein: 3g
Fat: 27g
Calories: 303

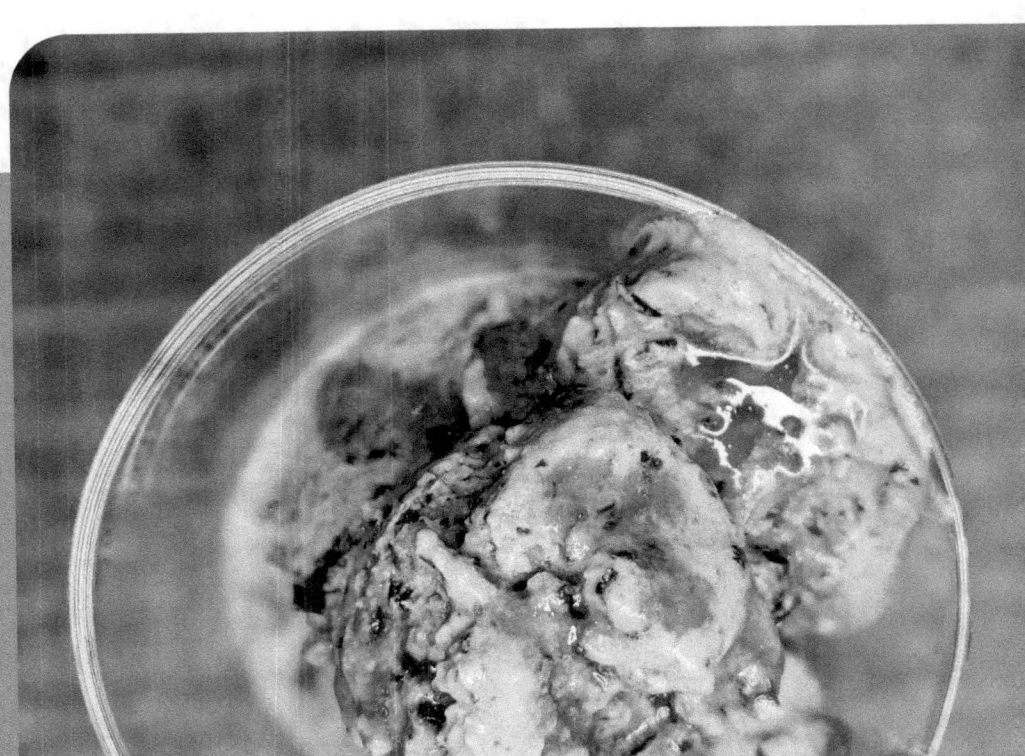

Quick & Simple Dairy-Free Berry Frozen Yogurt

Prep Time: 10 minutes

Cook Time: 0 minutes

Serves: 3

Difficulty Level: 1

Cost: $$

Ingredients:

- 1 cup frozen blueberries
- 1 cup frozen blackberries
- ½ cup full-fat unsweetened coconut milk
- 2 tsp monk fruit sweetener
- 1 tsp pure vanilla extract

Directions:

1. Add all ingredients to a blender and blend until creamy.
2. Enjoy right away.

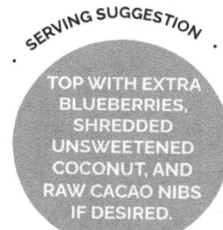

SERVING SUGGESTION

TOP WITH EXTRA BLUEBERRIES, SHREDDED UNSWEETENED COCONUT, AND RAW CACAO NIBS IF DESIRED.

Nutritional Information:

Carbs: 14g

Fiber: 4g

Net Carbs: 10g

Protein: 1g

Fat: 2g

Calories: 72

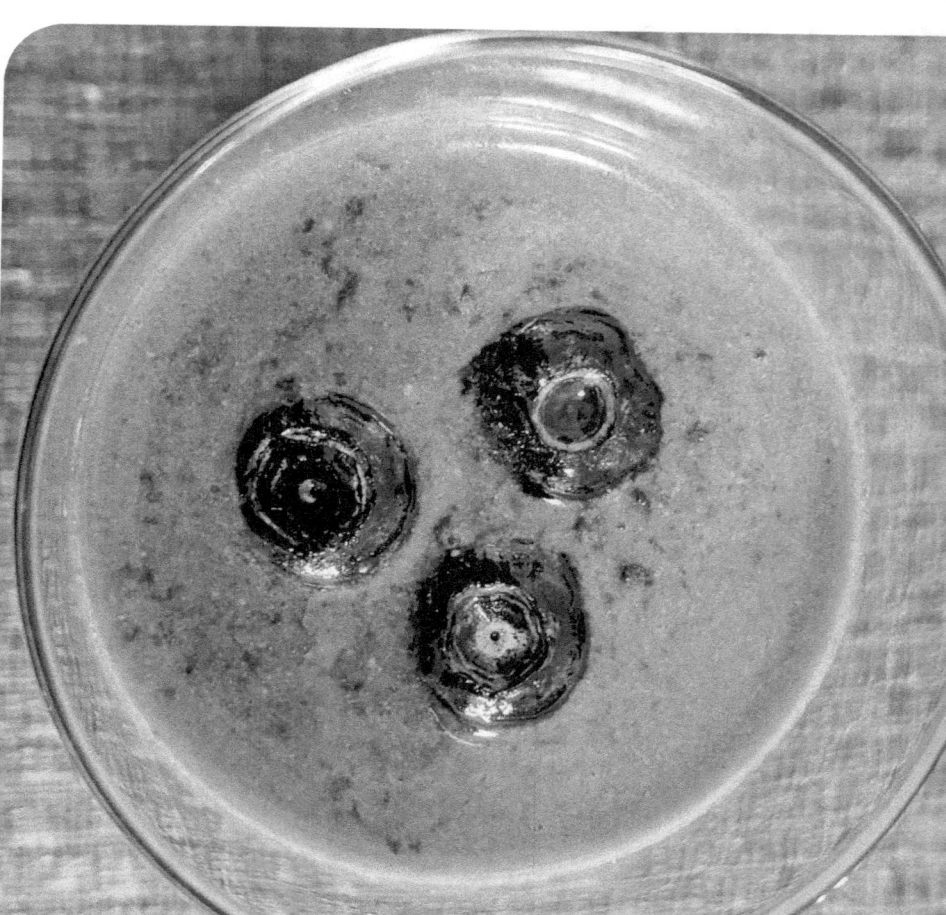

Oranges & Cream Ice Cream

Prep Time: 5 minutes
Cook Time: 0 minutes
Serves: 3
Difficulty Level: 1
Cost: $$

Ingredients:

- 1 orange, peeled and sliced
- 1 avocado, pitted and cubed
- ¼ cup full-fat unsweetened coconut milk
- 1 tsp pure vanilla extract
- Zero carb sweetener of choice
- **For topping:** Shredded coconut, raw cacao nibs

Directions:

1. Add all ingredients to a blender or food processor and blend until creamy.
2. Top with desired toppings and enjoy!

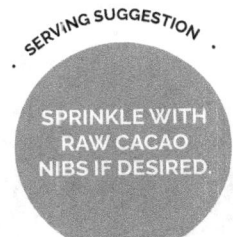

SERVING SUGGESTION

SPRINKLE WITH RAW CACAO NIBS IF DESIRED.

Nutritional Information:
Carbs: 13g
Fiber: 6g
Net Carbs: 7g
Protein: 2g
Fat: 14g
Calories: 180

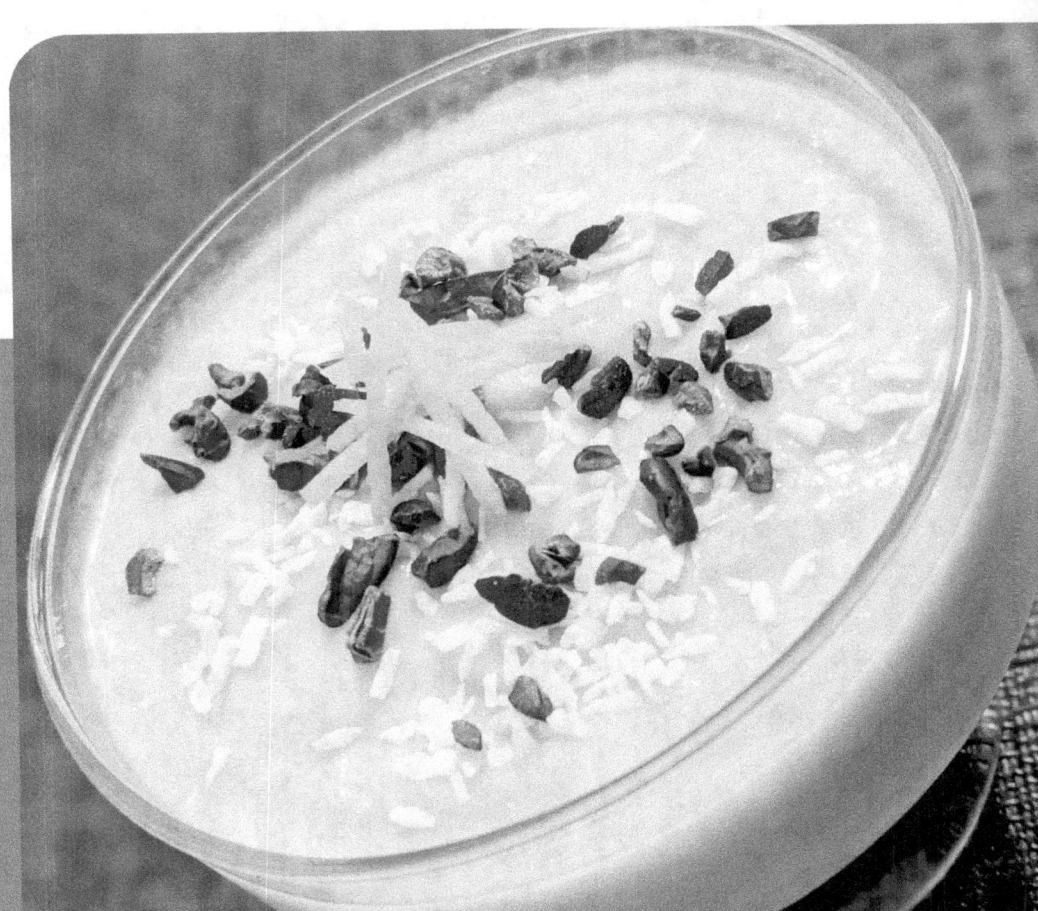

Toasted Coconut Dairy Free Milkshake

Prep Time: 5 minutes
Cook Time: 0 minutes
Serves: 2
Difficulty Level: 1
Cost: $$

Ingredients:

- 1 cup full-fat unsweetened coconut milk
- 1 tbsp shredded toasted coconut
- 1 tbsp coconut butter
- 1 tsp pure vanilla extract
- Low carb sweetener of choice

Directions:

1. Add all ingredients to a blender and blend until creamy.
2. Enjoy!

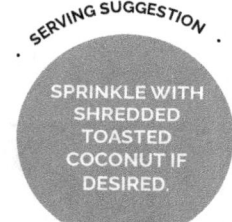

SERVING SUGGESTION

SPRINKLE WITH SHREDDED TOASTED COCONUT IF DESIRED.

Nutritional Information:
Carbs: 5g
Fiber: 3g
Net Carbs: 2g
Protein: 2g
Fat: 16g
Calories: 168

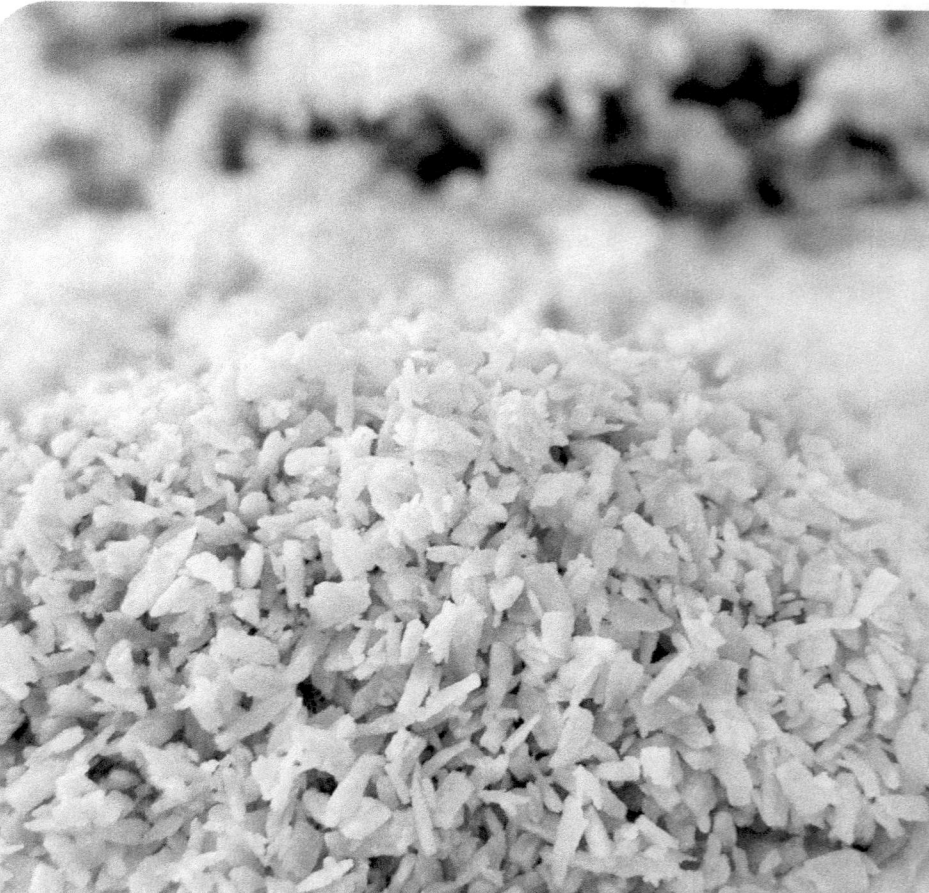

Creamy Vanilla Almond Dairy Free Milkshake

Prep Time: 5 minutes
Cook Time: 0 minutes
Serves: 2
Difficulty Level: 1
Cost: $$

Ingredients:

- ½ cup unsweetened almond milk
- ½ cup unsweetened coconut milk
- 1 tsp pure vanilla extract
- 1 tbsp almond butter
- 1 handful of ice cubes
- Low carb sweetener of choice

Directions:

1. Add all ingredients to a blender and blend until creamy.
2. Enjoy!

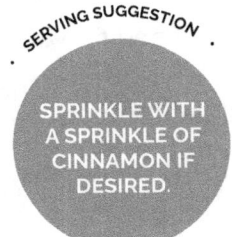

SERVING SUGGESTION

SPRINKLE WITH A SPRINKLE OF CINNAMON IF DESIRED.

Nutritional Information:
Carbs: 6g
Fiber: 2g
Net Carbs: 4g
Protein: 3g
Fat: 20g
Calories: 203

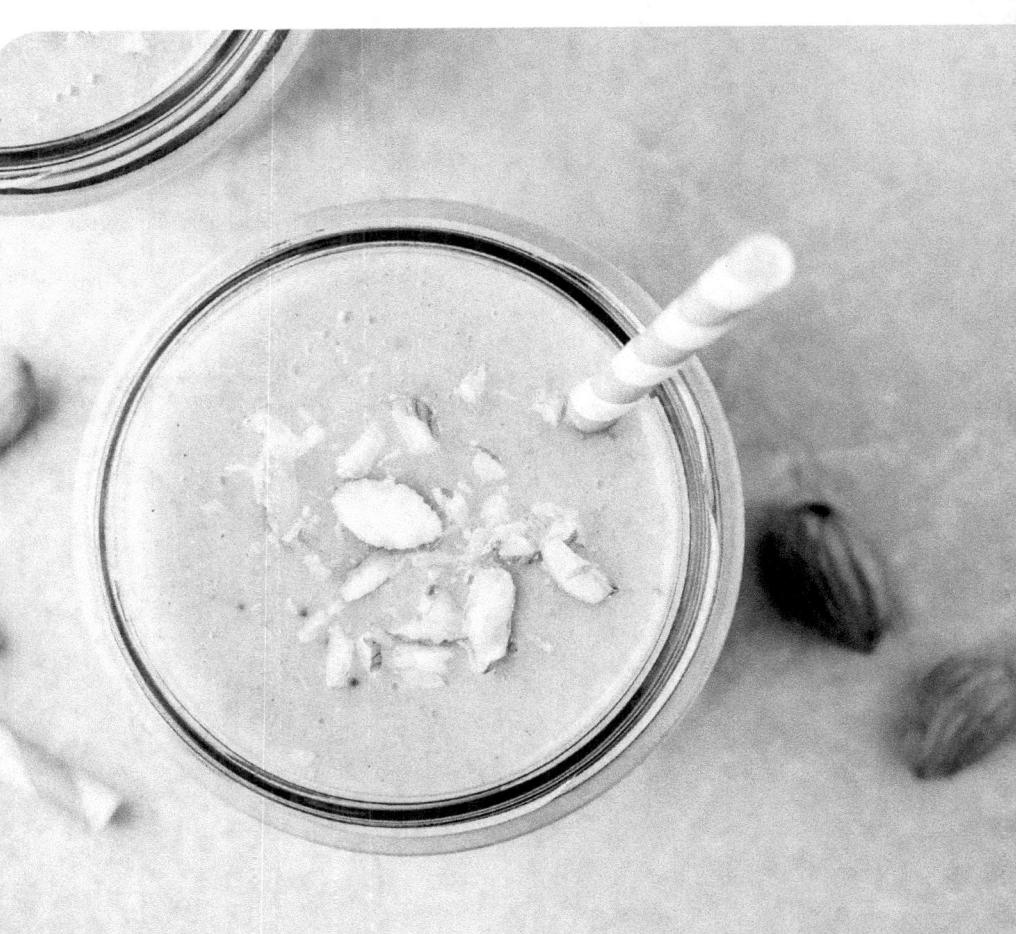

Decadent Blender Cinnamon Pecan Brownies

Prep Time: 15 minutes
Cook Time: 15-20 minutes
Serves: 10
Difficulty Level: 2
Cost: $$

Ingredients:

- 1 cup almond flour
- ½ cup unsweetened cacao powder
- 2 eggs
- ¼ cup coconut oil, melted
- 1 tsp pure vanilla extract
- ¼ cup pecans, chopped
- 1 tsp ground cinnamon
- ½ tsp liquid stevia

Directions:

1. Start by preheating the oven to 350 degrees F and line a brownie pan with parchment paper.
2. Add all ingredients to a blender and blend until smooth.
3. Pour into the lined brownie pan and bake for 15-20 minutes or until a toothpick inserted into the center comes out clean.
4. Cool and slice into brownies.
5. Store leftovers in an airtight container in the fridge.

· SERVING SUGGESTION ·

TOP WITH FULL-FAT UNSWEETENED COCONUT WHIPPED CREAM IF DESIRED.

Nutritional Information:
Carbs: 10g
Fiber: 6g
Net Carbs: 4g
Protein: 5g
Fat: 15g
Calories: 155

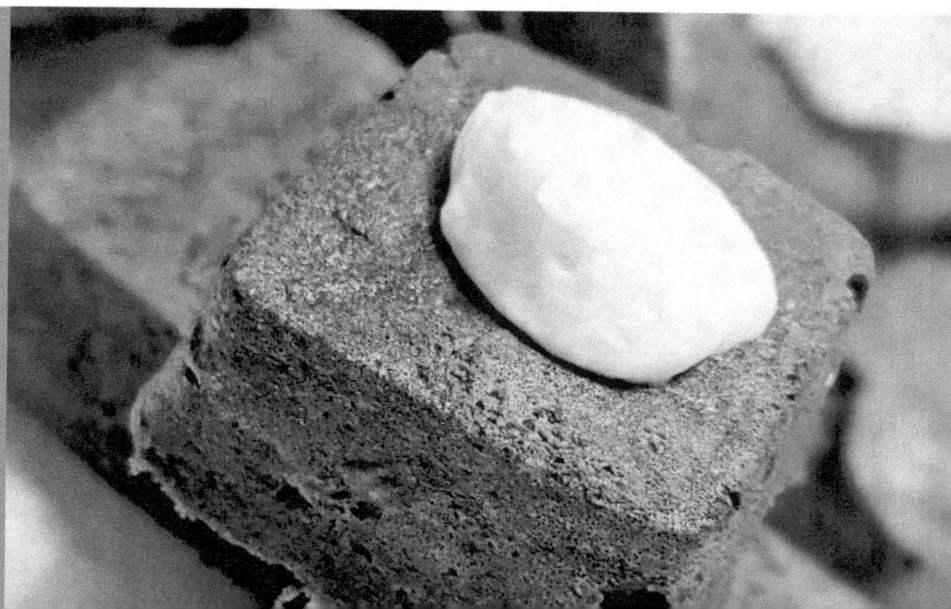

Chocolate Coffee Dairy Free Milkshake

Prep Time: 5 minutes
Cook Time: 0 minutes
Serves: 2
Difficulty Level: 1
Cost: $$

Ingredients:

- 1 cup brewed coffee, chilled
- ½ cup full-fat unsweetened coconut milk
- 1 tbsp unsweetened cacao powder
- 1 tbsp almond butter
- 1 tsp ground cinnamon

Directions:

1. Add all ingredients to a blender and blend until smooth.
2. Enjoy!

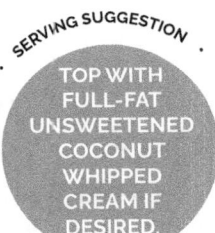

SERVING SUGGESTION

TOP WITH FULL-FAT UNSWEETENED COCONUT WHIPPED CREAM IF DESIRED.

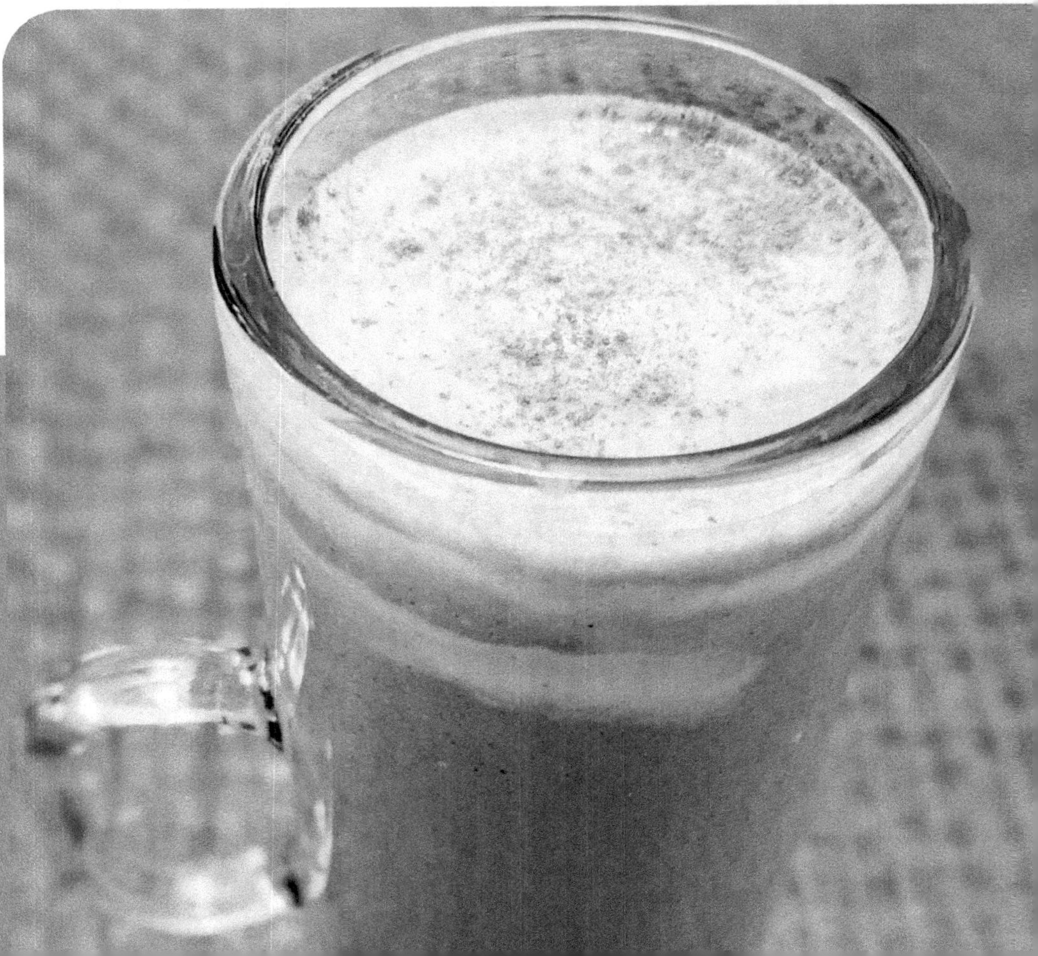

Nutritional Information:
Carbs: 11g
Fiber: 6g
Net Carbs: 5g
Protein: 5g
Fat: 21g
Calories: 216

Almond Cinnamon Cookies

Prep Time: 15 minutes
Cook Time: 10-15 minutes
Serves: 12
Difficulty Level: 2
Cost: $$

Ingredients:

- 2 eggs
- 1 tsp pure vanilla extract
- ¼ cup coconut oil, melted
- 1 cup almond flour
- ¼ cup erythritol
- 1 tsp ground cinnamon

Directions:

1. Start by preheating the oven to 350 degrees F and line a cookie sheet with parchment paper.

2. Add the eggs to a mixing bowl and whisk well. Add the vanilla and melted coconut oil and whisk again.

3. Add in the remaining ingredients and mix until clump free.

4. Drop by the rounded tablespoon onto the baking sheet and bake for 10-15 minutes.

SERVING SUGGESTION

WHISK TOGETHER EXTRA MONK FRUIT SWEETENER AND GROUND CINNAMON AND SPRINKLE ON TOP OF EACH COOKIE IF DESIRED.

Nutritional Information:
Carbs: 6g
Fiber: 0g
Net Carbs:
Protein: 1g
Fat: 6g
Calories: 64

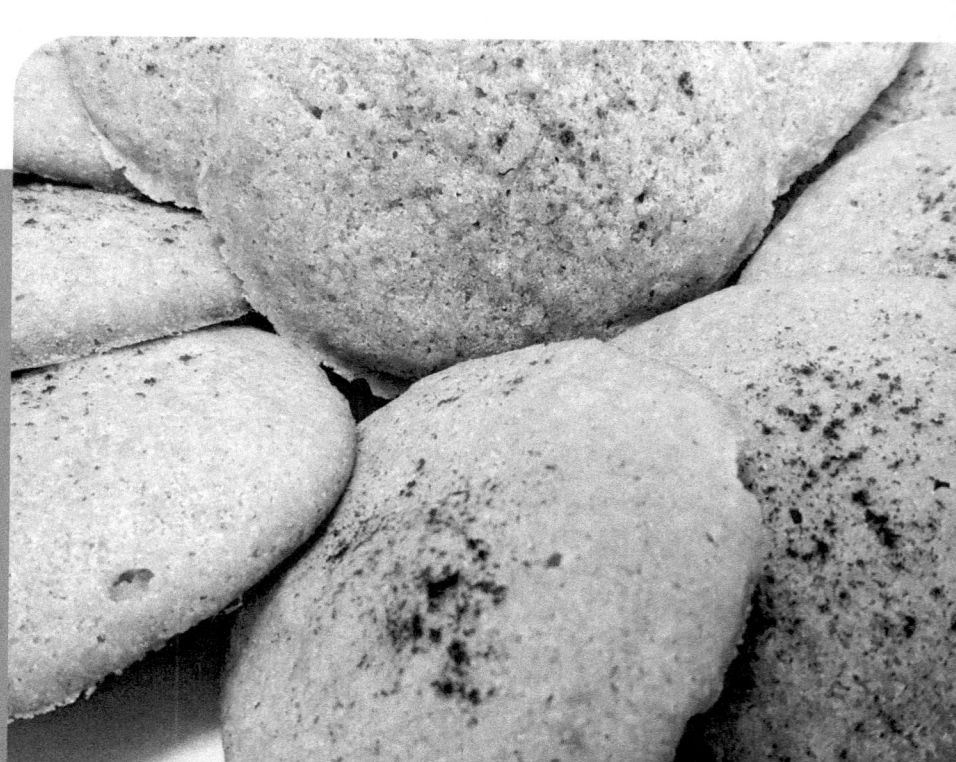

Chocolate Mousse

Prep Time: 10 minutes
Cook Time: 0 minutes
Serves: 3
Difficulty Level: 1
Cost: $

SERVING SUGGESTION

SERVE WITH SHREDDED UNSWEETENED COCONUT AND RAW CACAO NIBS IF DESIRED.

Ingredients:

- 1 cup full-fat unsweetened coconut milk
- 2 tbsp unsweetened cacao powder
- 1 tsp ground cinnamon
- 1 tsp pure vanilla extract
- 6 drops liquid stevia

Directions:

1. Add all ingredients to a mixing bowl and using a hand held mixer, mix until creamy.
2. Set in the fridge for 1 hour before serving.

Nutritional Information:
Carbs: 12g
Fiber: 6g
Net Carbs: 6g
Protein: 5g
Fat: 22g
Calories: 223

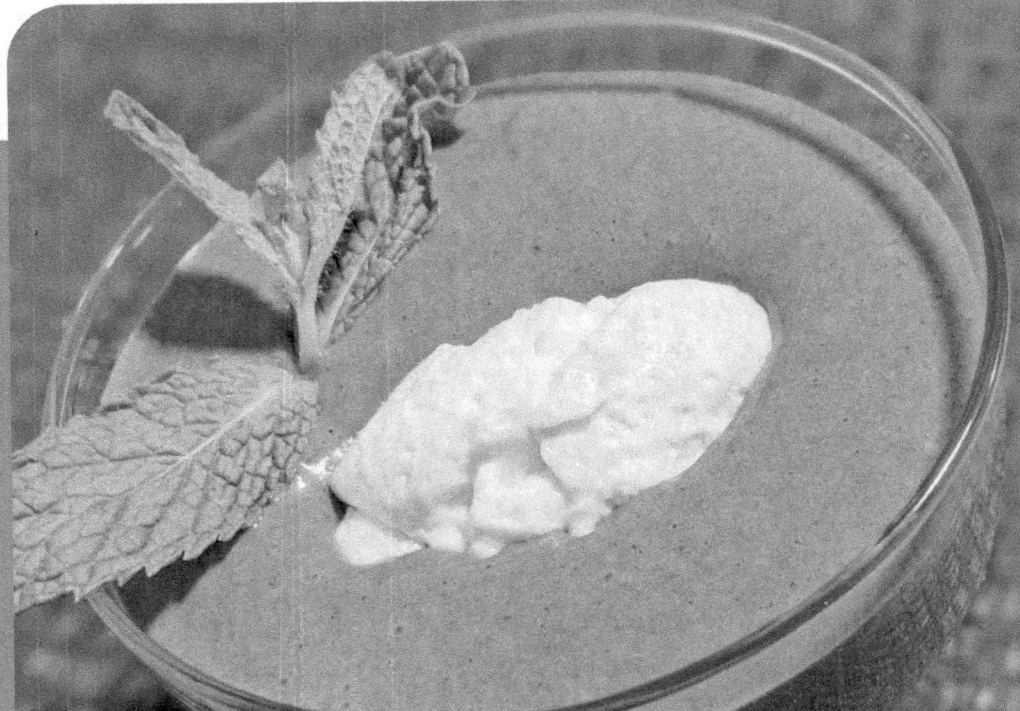

Decadent Raw Brownies

Prep Time: 10 minutes
+ chilling time
Cook Time: 0 minutes
Serves: 12
Difficulty Level: 2
Cost: $$

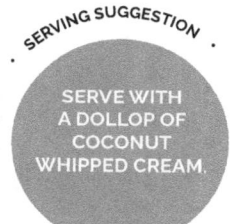

· SERVING SUGGESTION ·

SERVE WITH
A DOLLOP OF
COCONUT
WHIPPED CREAM.

Ingredients:

- 2 cups almond flour
- 2 cups almond butter
- ½ cup unsweetened cacao powder
- 1 tsp ground cinnamon
- 1 tsp pure vanilla extract
- ½ tsp sea salt
- ½ cup monk fruit maple syrup

Directions:

1. Add all ingredients to a blender and blend until smooth.
2. Pour into a parchment-lined brownie pan and press flat.
3. Set in the freezer for 30 minutes.
4. Once chilled, slice into brownies and store leftovers in an airtight container in the fridge.

Nutritional Information:
Carbs: 10g
Fiber: 5g
Net Carbs: 5g
Protein: 4g
Fat: 7g
Calories: 83

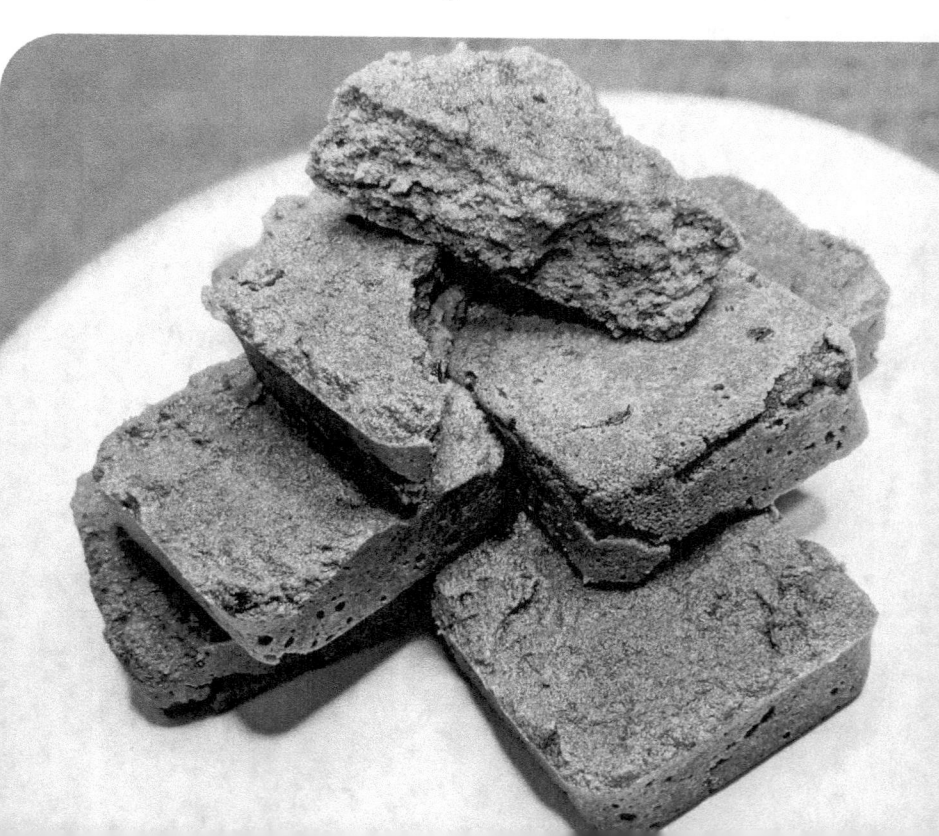

Coconut Whipped Cream

Prep Time: 15 minutes
Cook Time: 0 minutes
Serves: 8
Difficulty Level: 1
Cost: $

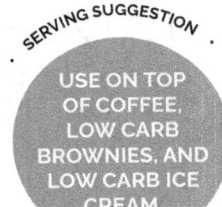

SERVING SUGGESTION

USE ON TOP OF COFFEE, LOW CARB BROWNIES, AND LOW CARB ICE CREAM.

Ingredients:

- 2 cups full-fat unsweetened coconut milk
- 1 tsp pure vanilla extract
- 2 tbsp erythritol

Directions:

1. Start by adding a freezer-safe mixing bowl to the freezer for 10 minutes.
2. Add all ingredients to the mixing bowl and using a handheld mixer, whip until a whip-cream like consistency forms.
3. Enjoy right away!

Nutritional Information:
Carbs: 7g
Fiber: 1g
Net Carbs: 6g
Protein: 1g
Fat: 14g
Calories: 140

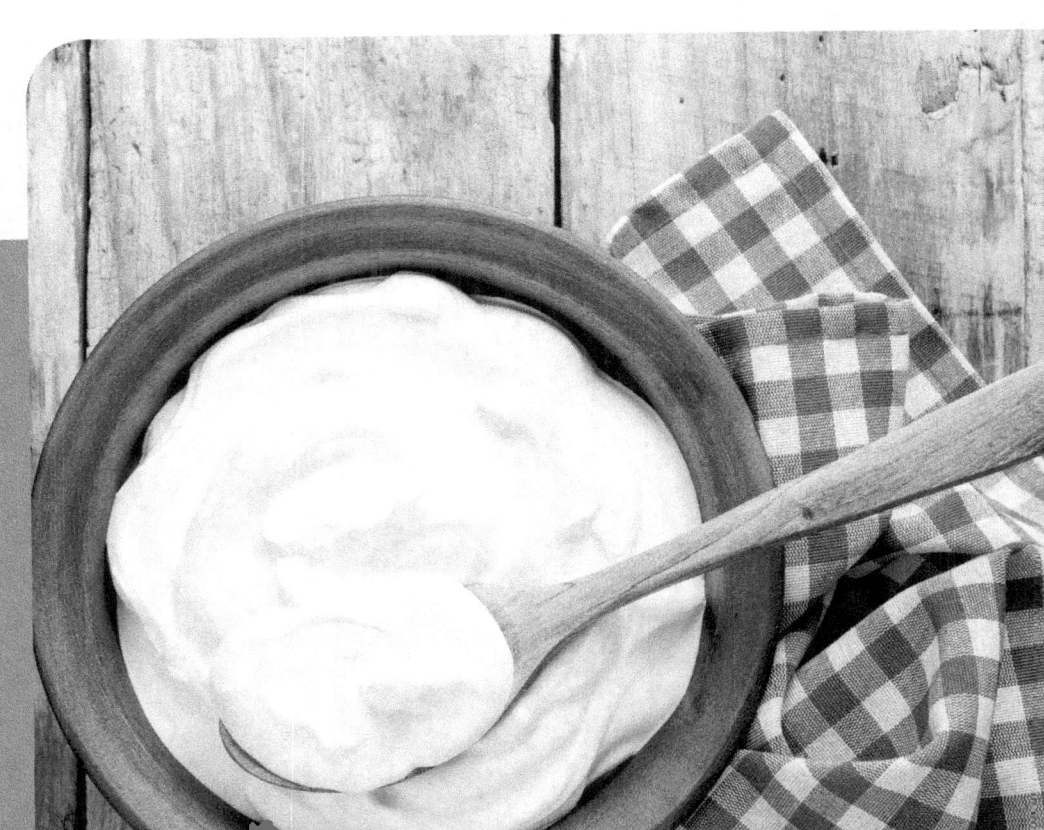

Key Lime Pie Pudding

Prep Time: 15 minutes + chilling time

Cook Time: 0 minutes

Serves: 5

Difficulty Level: 1

Cost: $$

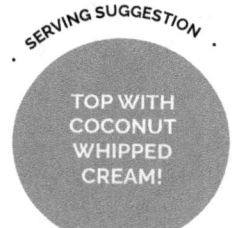

SERVING SUGGESTION

TOP WITH COCONUT WHIPPED CREAM!

Ingredients:

- 2 cups unsweetened coconut milk yogurt
- 1 ripe avocado, pitted and sliced
- 2 tbsp freshly squeezed lime juice
- 2 tbsp erythritol or low carb sweetener of choice
- ¼ cup almonds, crushed for serving

Directions:

1. Add all the ingredients to a blender and blend until smooth.
2. Add the crushed almonds to the base of five serving jars or bowls and split the key lime pie mixture between the cups, adding on top of the almonds. Chill in the fridge for 1 hour before serving.
3. Enjoy!

Nutritional Information:

Carbs: 13g

Fiber: 5g

Net Carbs: 8g

Protein: 2g

Fat: 12g

Calories: 130

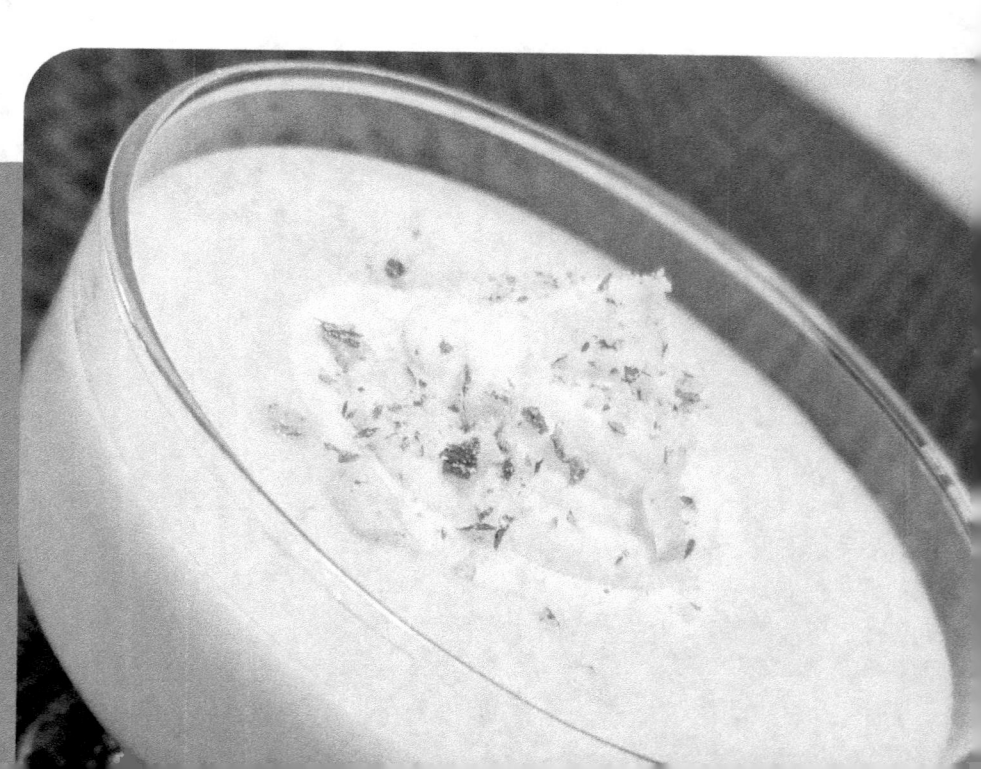

Coconut Slush Dessert

Prep Time: 5 minutes

Cook Time: 0 minutes

Serves: 1

Difficulty Level: 1

Cost: $

Ingredients:

- 1 cup coconut cream
- ½ cup sugar-free pineapple sparkling water
- Juice of 1 lemon
- Handful of ice
- Shredded coconut, for topping (optional)

Directions:

1. Place all of the ingredients except for the shredded coconut into a high-speed blender and blend until smooth.

2. Top with shredded coconut, if desired.

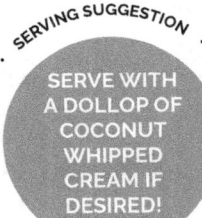

SERVING SUGGESTION

SERVE WITH A DOLLOP OF COCONUT WHIPPED CREAM IF DESIRED!

Nutritional Information:

Carbs: 13g

Fiber: 5g

Net Carbs: 8g

Protein: 5g

Fat: 57g

Calories: 552

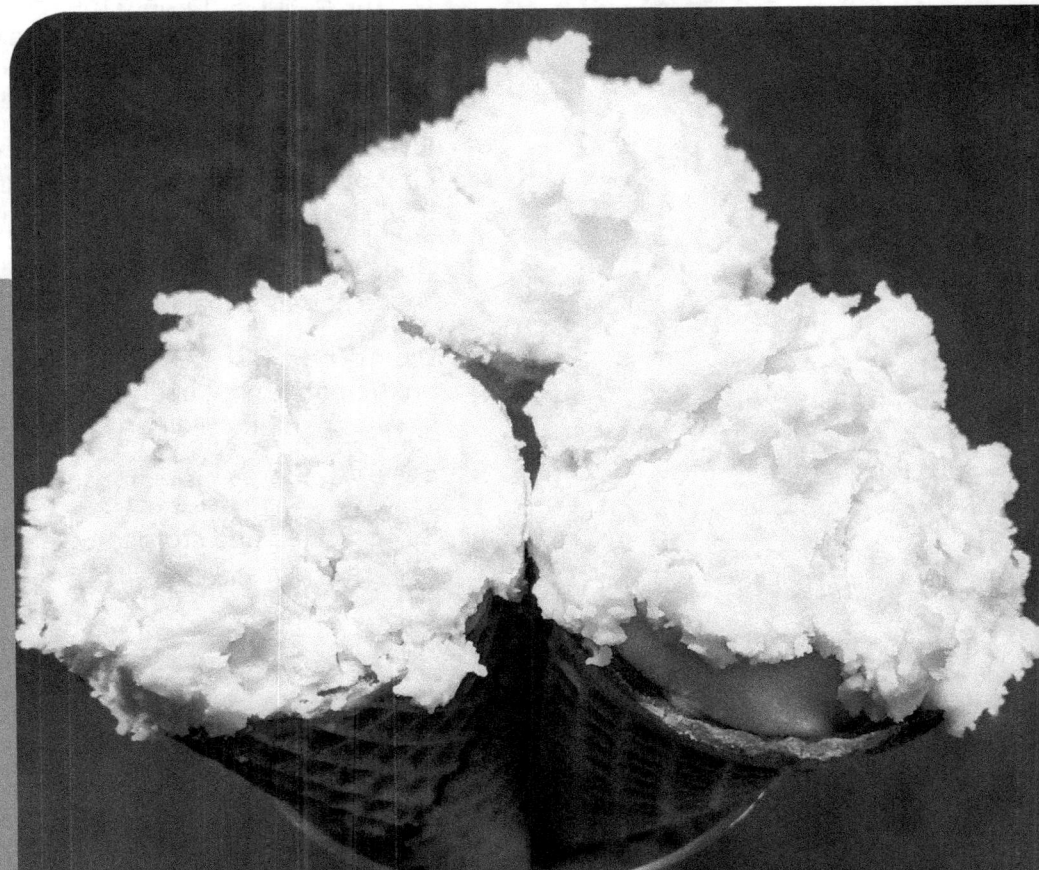

Chocolate Covered Candied Bacon

Prep Time: 15 minutes
Cook Time: 15-25 minutes
Serves: 4
Difficulty Level: 2
Cost: $$

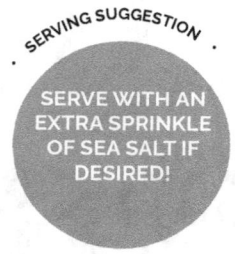

SERVING SUGGESTION

SERVE WITH AN EXTRA SPRINKLE OF SEA SALT IF DESIRED!

Ingredients:

- 6 slices of uncured bacon
- ½ cup sugar-free maple syrup
- ½ tsp. pure vanilla extract
- ¼ cup sugar-free dark chocolate chips
- 2 Tbsp. coconut oil
- ½ tsp. sea salt + more for serving

Directions:

1. Start by preheating the oven to 350 degrees Fahrenheit and lining a baking sheet with parchment paper.

2. Combine the maple syrup, vanilla and ½ tsp. salt in a small bowl and whisk to combine.

3. Dip the bacon strips into the mixture coating both sides and place on the parchment lined baking sheet.

4. Bake for 15-25 minutes or until the bacon is crispy.

5. Five minutes before the bacon is done cooking, place the chocolate chips and coconut oil into a small stockpot over low heat and whisk until melted. Remove from heat.

6. Once the bacon is cooked, allow it to cool and then cut into 1-inch squares, making 28 total.

7. Dip the bacon squares into the chocolate and place back on the parchment lined baking sheet, or if needed into a smaller parchment lined container.

8. Refrigerate for 30 minutes to set.

9. Serve chilled and store leftovers in the fridge.

Nutritional Information:

Carbs: 9g

Fiber: 2g

Net Carbs: 7g

Protein: 12g

Fat: 25g

Calories: 284

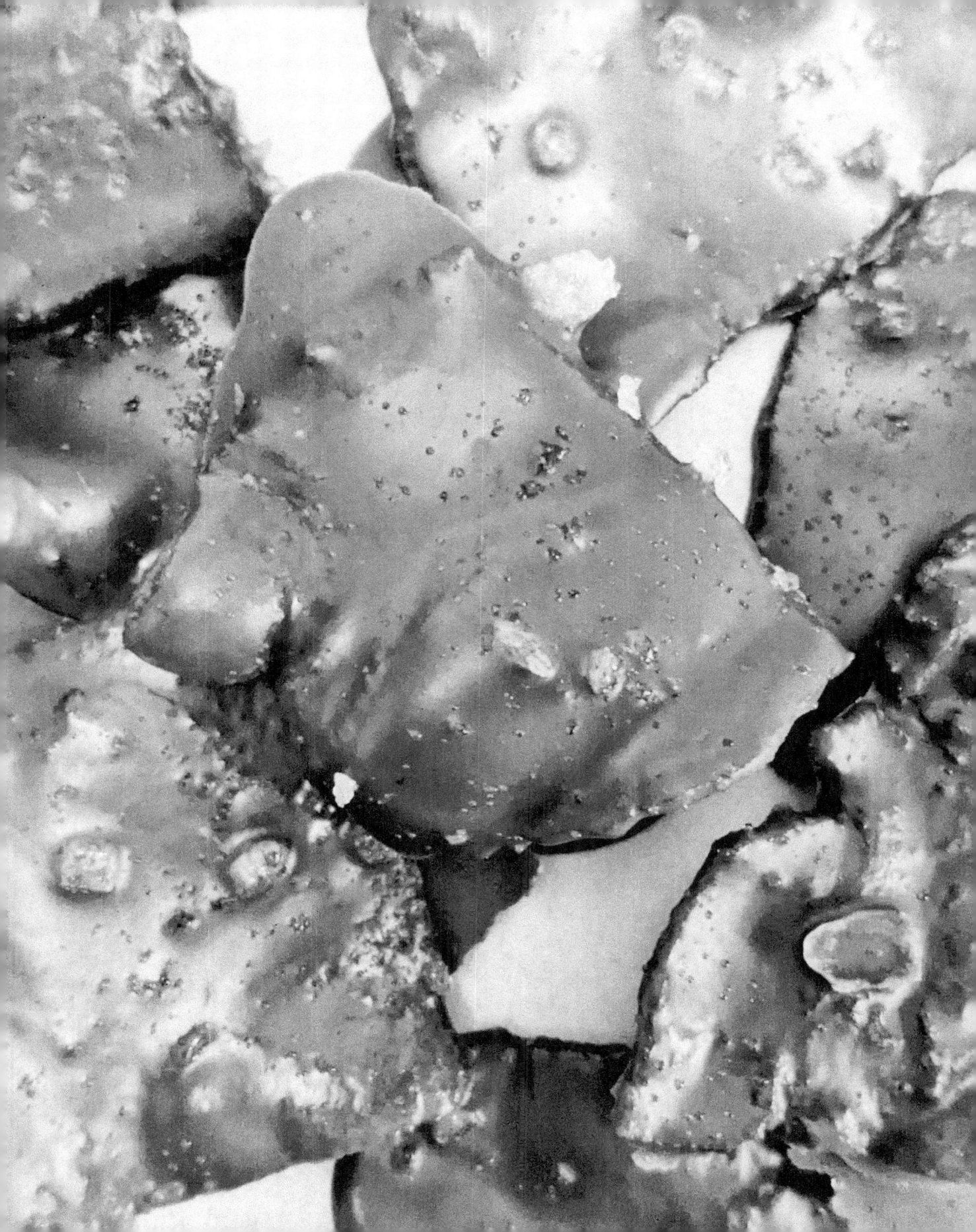

Belgian Chocolate Mousse

Prep Time: 10 minutes
Cook Time: 5 minutes
Serves: 3
Difficulty Level: 1
Cost: $

SERVING SUGGESTION

SPRINKLE WITH SHREDDED TOASTED COCONUT IF DESIRED.

Ingredients:

- 1 can full-fat coconut milk
- 3 Tbsp. raw cocoa powder
- 3 eggs
- Mint leaf, for garnish (optional)

Directions:

1. Refrigerate the coconut milk the night before you want to make this recipe. The next morning, remove only the hardened part of the milk and add this to a stockpot.

2. Add the eggs and cocoa powder and whisk over low heat until combined and the coconut cream has softened.

3. Chill before serving, and then serve in 3 individual dessert bowls.

4. Add a mint leaf as garnish, if desired.

Nutritional Information:
Carbs: 8g
Fiber: 4g
Net Carbs: 4g
Protein: 8g
Fat: 24g
Calories: 259

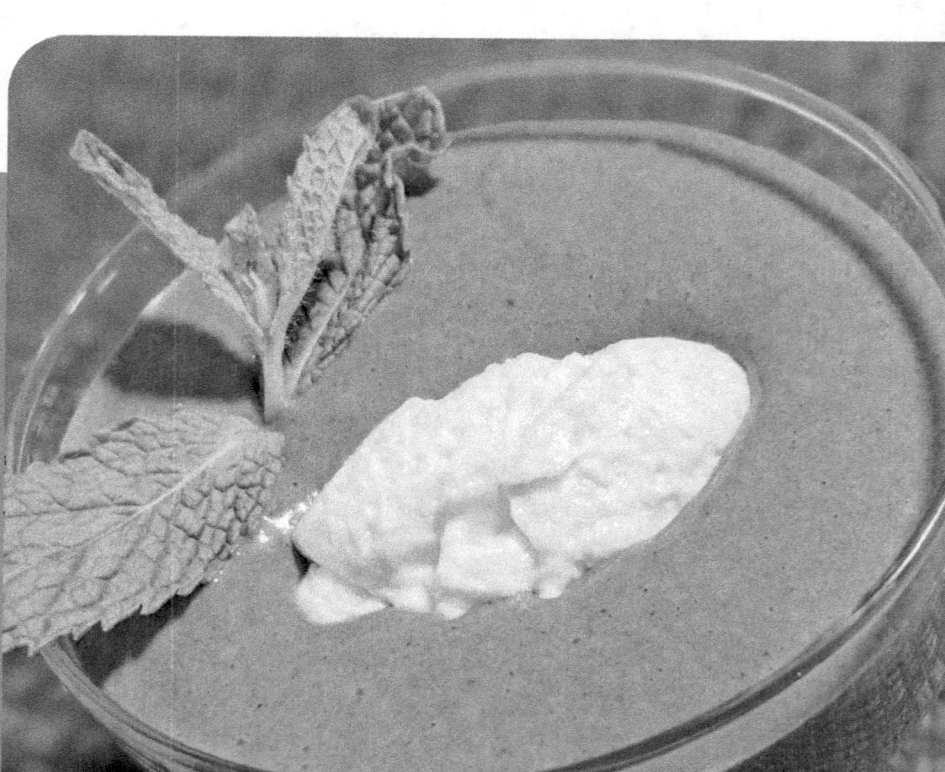

Icelandic Cocoa Soup

Prep Time: 5 minutes
Cook Time: 5 minutes
Serves: 4
Difficulty Level: 1
Cost: $$

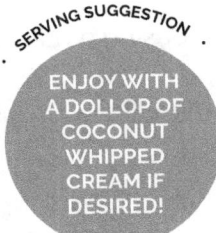

SERVING SUGGESTION

ENJOY WITH
A DOLLOP OF
COCONUT
WHIPPED
CREAM IF
DESIRED!

Ingredients:

- 2 Tbsp. raw cocoa powder
- ½ tsp. ground cinnamon
- 2 tsp. pure vanilla extract
- 2 cups water
- 3 cups coconut milk
- 1 drop liquid vanilla stevia
- 1 Tbsp. gluten-free cornstarch

Directions:

1. Pour the water and coconut milk into a saucepan, add the cinnamon and cocoa powder, and whisk.

2. Add the vanilla extract, cornstarch, and stevia.

3. Stir over low heat until warmed throughout, being careful not to burn the milk.

Nutritional Information:

Carbs: 14g

Fiber: 5g

Net Carbs: 9g

Protein: 5g

Fat: 43g

Calories: 434

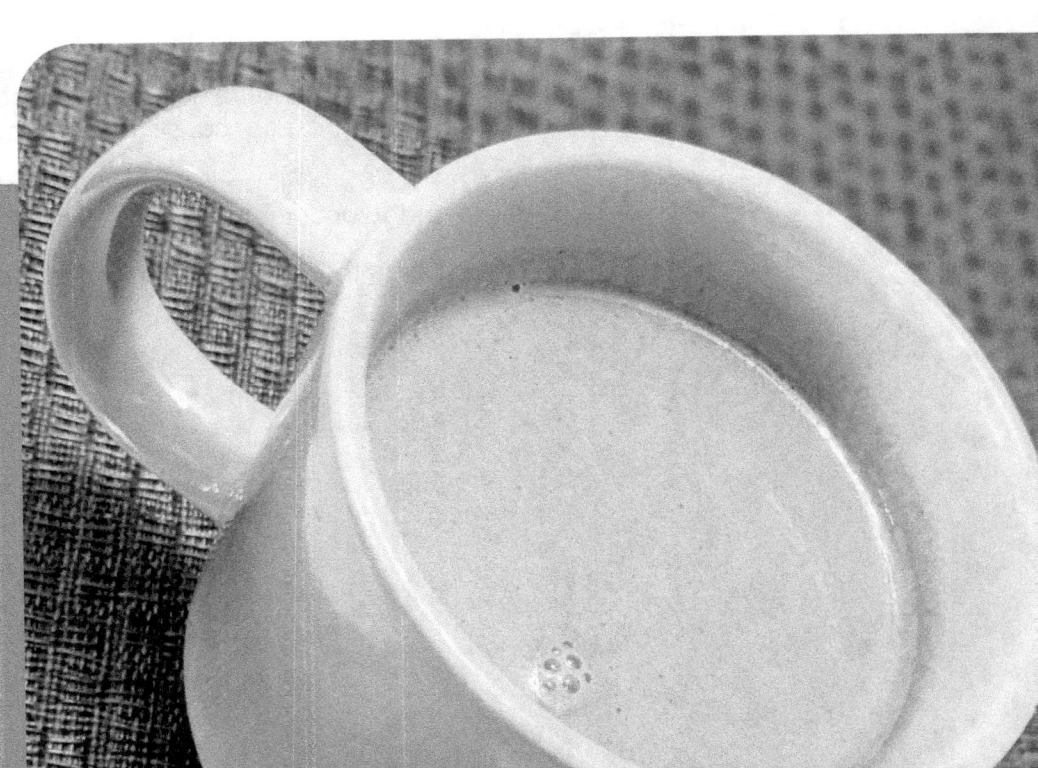

Coconut Brownie Sundae

Prep Time: 15 minutes
Cook Time: 25-30 minutes
Serves: 8
Difficulty Level: 2
Cost: $

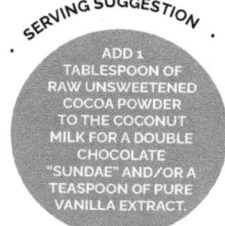

SERVING SUGGESTION

ADD 1 TABLESPOON OF RAW UNSWEETENED COCOA POWDER TO THE COCONUT MILK FOR A DOUBLE CHOCOLATE "SUNDAE" AND/OR A TEASPOON OF PURE VANILLA EXTRACT.

Ingredients:

- 2 Tbsp. coconut flour, sifted
- 3 Tbsp. raw unsweetened cocoa powder
- ½ cup coconut oil, melted
- 2 eggs
- 1 tsp. pure vanilla extract
- ¼ cup erythritol
- 2 cups full-fat unsweetened coconut milk (canned)

Directions:

1. Start by preheating the oven to 350°F and greasing a baking dish with coconut oil.

2. Add all of the ingredients, minus the coconut milk, to a food processor and blend until smooth.

3. Pour the batter into the greased baking dish and bake for 25-30 minutes or until a knife inserted into the center comes out clean.

4. While the brownies are cooking, add the solid part from the can of coconut milk to a food processor and process until a whipped cream consistency forms.

5. Pour the whipped coconut milk into a bowl and chill it in the fridge until the brownies are cooked.

6. Serve the brownies with the whipped coconut cream.

Nutritional Information:
Carbs: 12g
Fiber: 2g
Net Carbs: 10g
Protein: 3g
Fat: 28g
Calories: 266

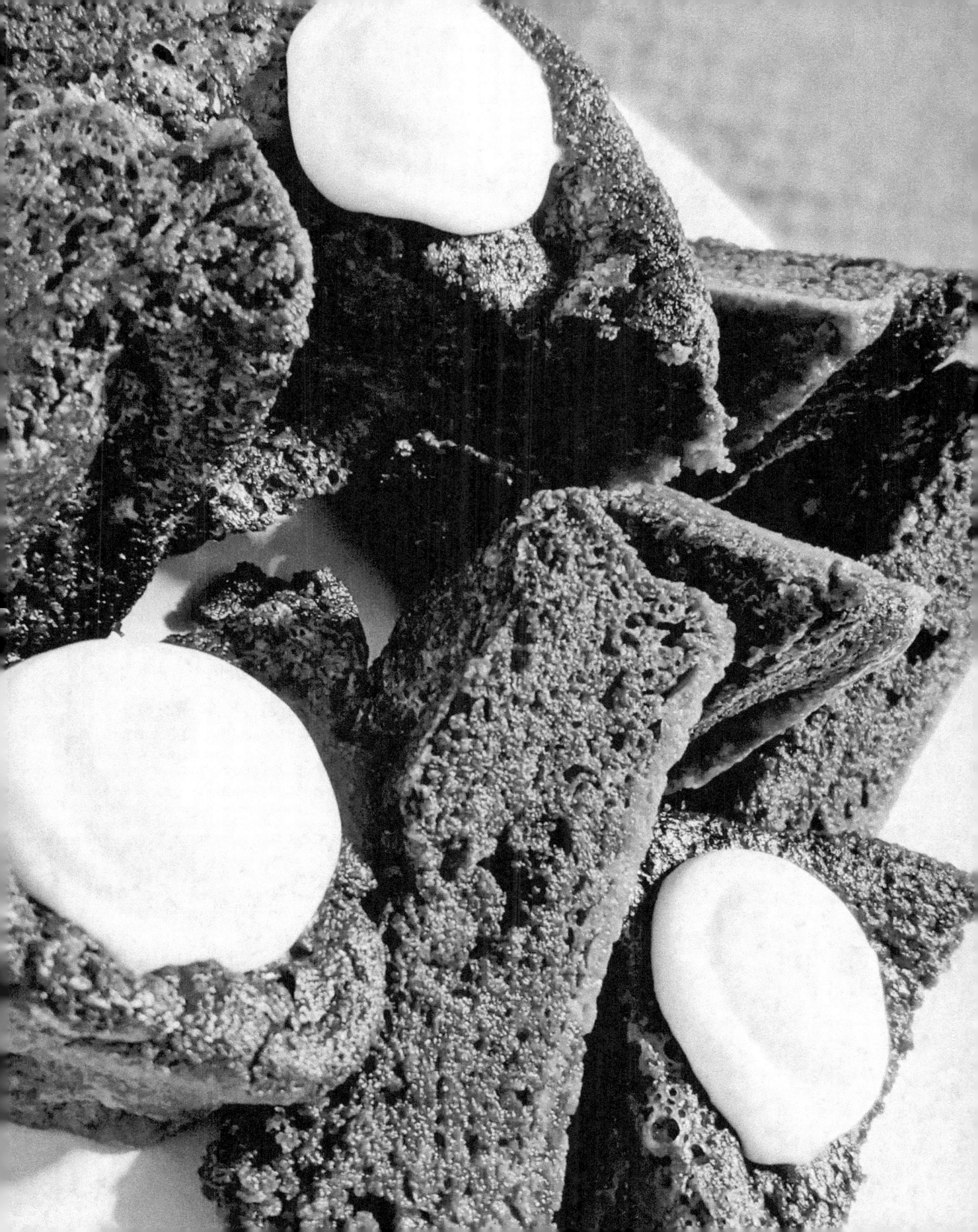

Devil's Food Donuts

Prep Time: 10 minutes
Cook Time: 15-20 minutes
Serves: 8
Difficulty Level: 2
Cost: $$

· SERVING SUGGESTION ·

SERVE WITH COCONUT WHIPPED CREAM AND A SLAB OF ALMOND BUTTER!

Ingredients:

- ¼ cup coconut flour, sifted
- 2 Tbsp. almond flour
- ¼ cup erythritol
- 1 tsp. baking powder
- ¼ cup raw unsweetened cocoa powder
- 5 eggs
- ¼ cup coconut oil, melted + more for greasing
- 1 tsp. pure vanilla extract

Directions:

1. Start by preheating the oven to 300°F and greasing a donut pan with coconut oil.

2. Add the coconut flour, erythritol, cocoa powder and baking powder to a large mixing bowl, and stir well.

3. Add in the remaining ingredients and whisk to combine.

4. Pour the batter into the donut pan and bake for 15-20 minutes or until the donuts are set and firm to touch.

5. Allow them to cool for 5 minutes before removing.

Nutritional Information:
Carbs: 15g
Fiber: 4g
Net Carbs: 11g
Protein: 5g
Fat: 12g
Calories: 146

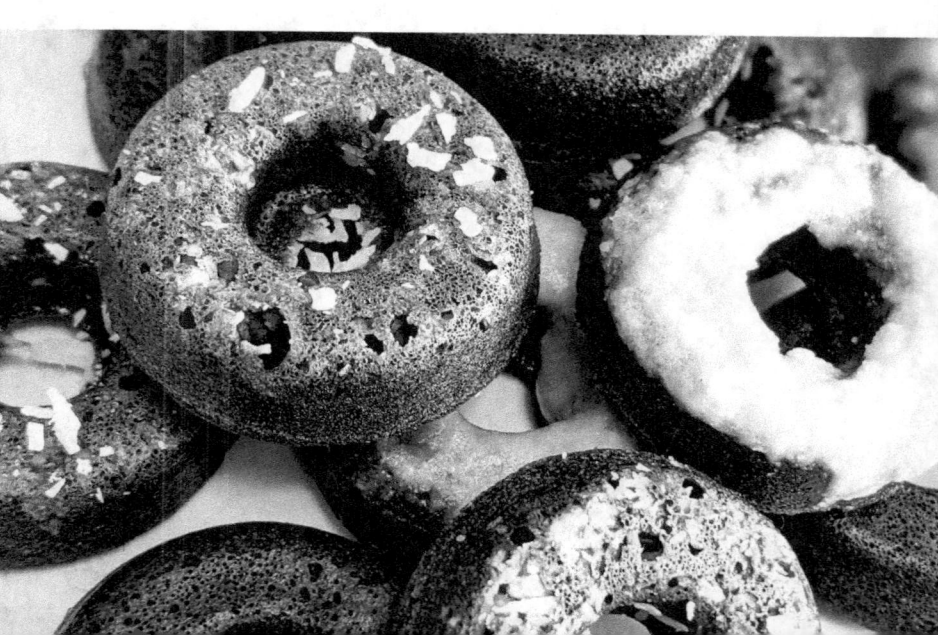

Drinks

Iced Coconut Cream Vegan Coffee

Prep Time: 10 minutes
Cook Time: 0 minutes
Serves: 1
Difficulty Level: 1
Cost: $

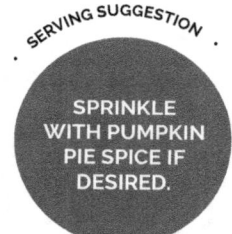

· SERVING SUGGESTION ·

SPRINKLE WITH PUMPKIN PIE SPICE IF DESIRED.

Ingredients:

- 1 cup brewed coffee, chilled
- ½ cup full-fat unsweetened coconut milk
- 1 tsp pure vanilla extract
- Zero carb sweetener of choice
- Ice cubes

Directions:

1. Start by adding ice cubes to a tall serving glass and add the chilled coffee and coconut milk, vanilla, and low carb sweetener of choice, and whisk well.

2. Enjoy!

Nutritional Information:

Carbs: 7g

Fiber: 3g

Net Carbs: 4g

Protein: 3g

Fat: 29g

Calories: 290

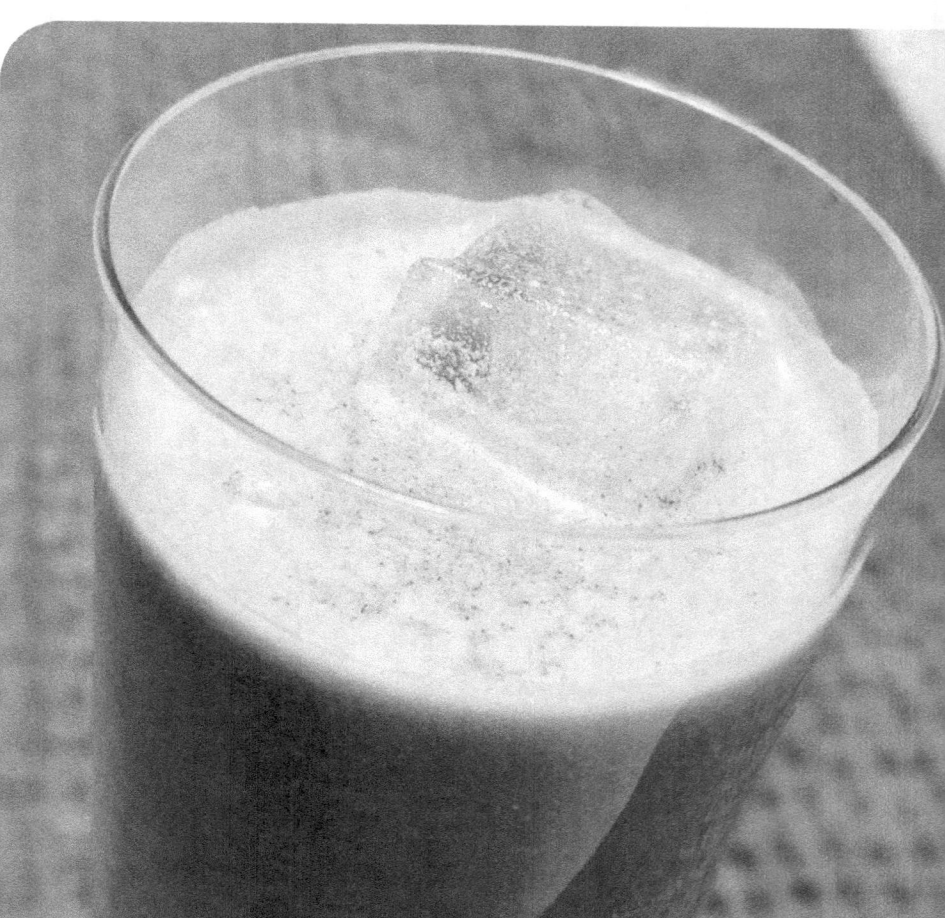

Dairy Free Mexican Hot Chocolate

Prep Time: 5 minutes
Cook Time: 5 minutes
Serves: 3
Difficulty Level: 1
Cost: $$

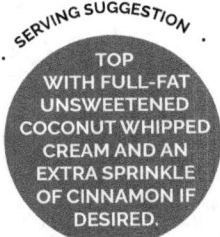

SERVING SUGGESTION

TOP WITH FULL-FAT UNSWEETENED COCONUT WHIPPED CREAM AND AN EXTRA SPRINKLE OF CINNAMON IF DESIRED.

Ingredients:

- 1 cup full-fat unsweetened coconut milk
- 2 tbsp raw cacao powder
- 1 tsp ground cinnamon
- ⅛ tsp cayenne pepper
- 3 drops liquid stevia
- 1 tsp pure vanilla extract

Directions:

1. Add all ingredients to a stock pot over low heat and whisk until warm.
2. Pour into your favorite mug and enjoy!

Nutritional Information:
Carbs: 12g
Fiber: 6g
Net Carbs: 6g
Protein: 5g
Fat: 22g
Calories: 224

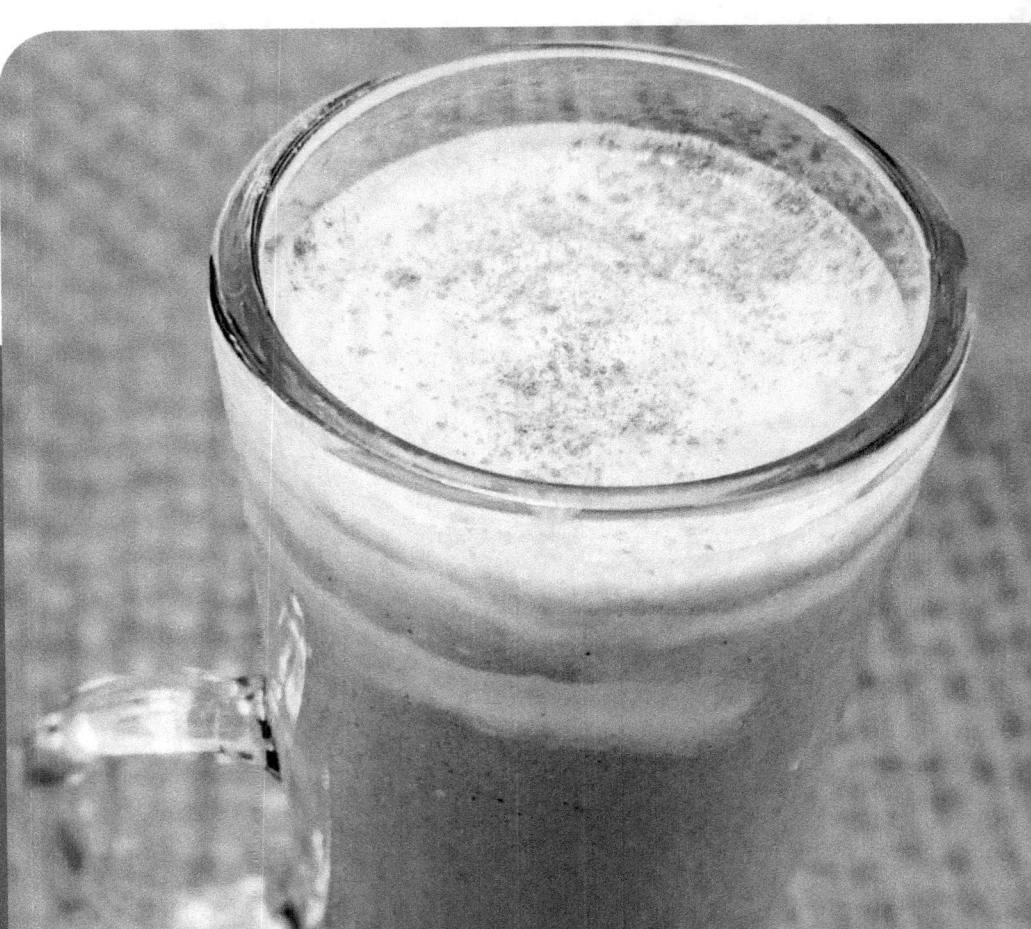

Homemade Cinnamon Almond Milk

Prep Time: 10 minutes
Cook Time: 0 minutes
Serves: 6
Difficulty Level: 1
Cost: $

Ingredients:

- 2 cups raw almonds
- 4 cups filtered water
- 1 tsp pure vanilla extract
- 1 ½ tsp ground cinnamon

Directions:

1. Add all ingredients to a blender and blend until smooth.
2. Strain through a cheesecloth and pour into a tall glass jar and store in the fridge.

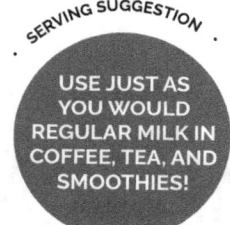

SERVING SUGGESTION

USE JUST AS YOU WOULD REGULAR MILK IN COFFEE, TEA, AND SMOOTHIES!

Nutritional Information:
Carbs: 7g
Fiber: 4g
Net Carbs: 3g
Protein: 7g
Fat: 16g
Calories: 187

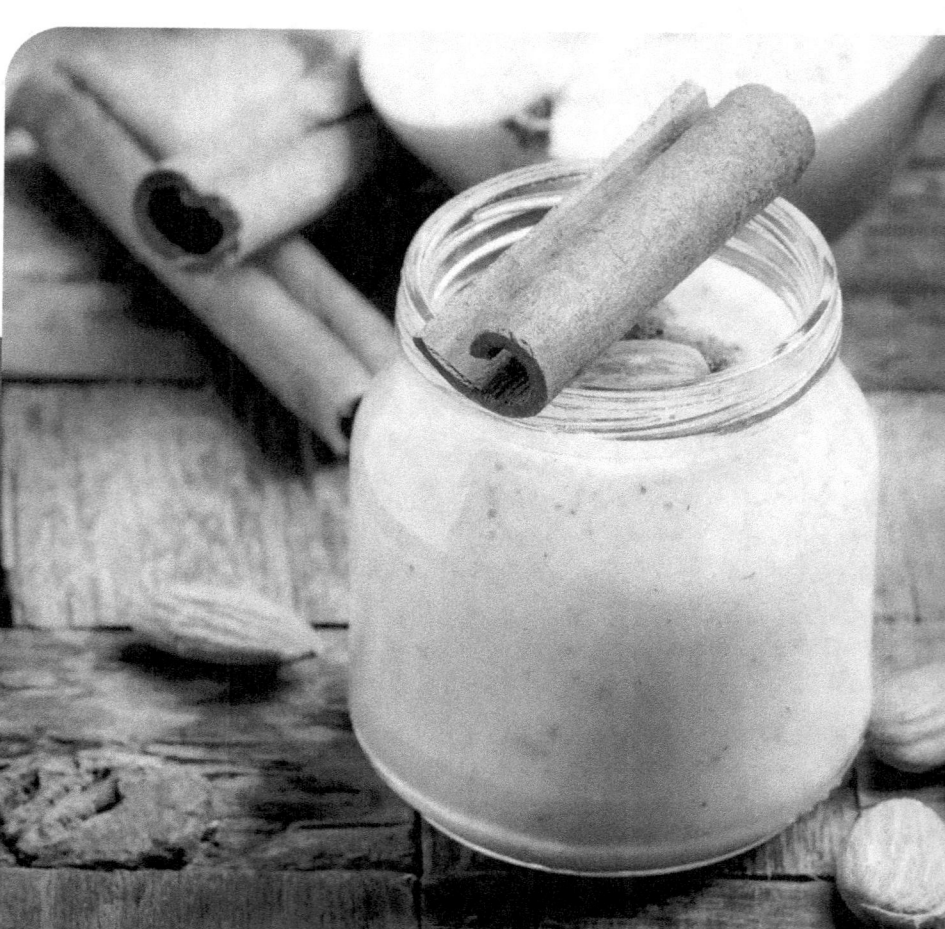

Iced Matcha Tea

Prep Time: 10 minutes
Cook Time: 0 minutes
Serves: 2
Difficulty Level: 1
Cost: $

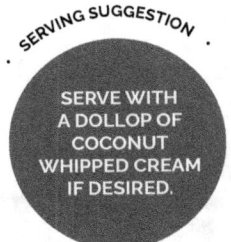

SERVING SUGGESTION

SERVE WITH A DOLLOP OF COCONUT WHIPPED CREAM IF DESIRED.

Ingredients:

- 1 cup unsweetened almond milk
- ¼ cup full-fat unsweetened coconut milk
- 1 tsp matcha powder
- Low carb sweetener of choice
- Ice

Directions:

1. Add all ingredients minus the ice to a blender and blend until smooth.
2. Serve over ice and enjoy right away.

Nutritional Information:
Carbs: 3g
Fiber: 1g
Net Carbs: 2g
Protein: 1g
Fat: 9g
Calories: 89

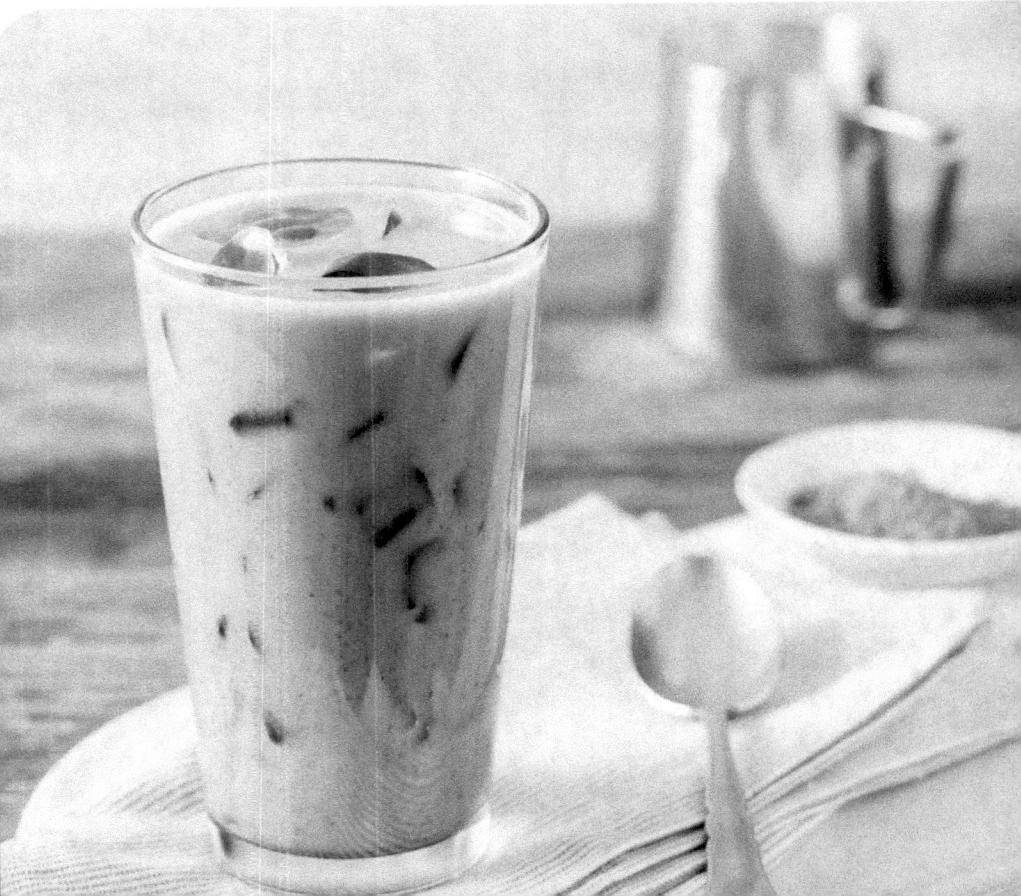

Lemon Iced Tea

Prep Time: 10 minutes
Cook Time: 0 minutes
Serves: 3
Difficulty Level: 1
Cost: $

SERVING SUGGESTION

SERVE WITH AN EXTRA SQUEEZE OF LEMON JUICE IF DESIRED.

Ingredients:

- 2 cups brewed black tea, chilled
- 2 tbsp freshly squeezed lime juice
- 3 drops liquid stevia
- Ice

Directions:

1. Add all ingredients minus the ice to a blender and blend for 30 seconds.

2. Pour into two serving glasses over ice.

3. Enjoy!

Nutritional Information:

Carbs: 1g
Fiber: 0
Net Carbs: 1g
Protein: 0
Fat: 0
Calories: 2

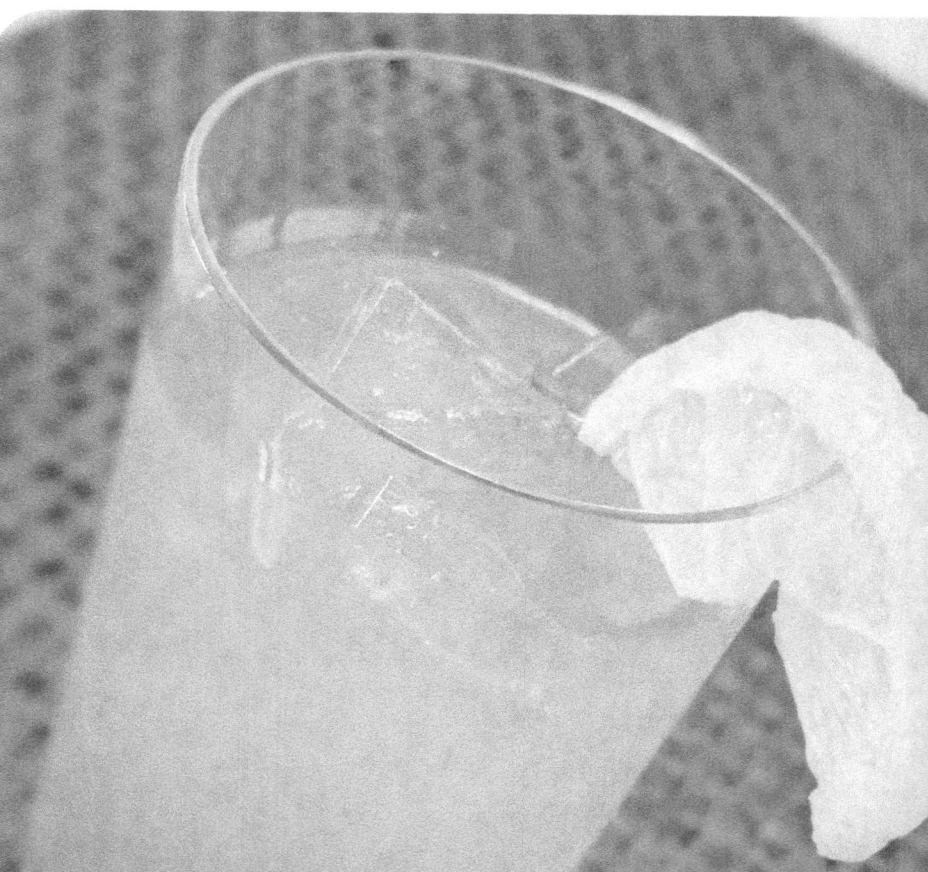

Keto Turmeric Latte

Prep Time: 10 minutes
Cook Time: 5 minutes
Serves: 2
Difficulty Level: 1
Cost: $$

Ingredients:

- 1 cup full-fat unsweetened coconut milk
- 1 tbsp coconut oil
- ½ tsp ground turmeric
- ½ tsp ground cinnamon
- 1 pinch of black pepper
- 3 drops of vanilla liquid stevia (or whatever one serving is depending on your liquid stevia)

Directions:

1. Add all ingredients to a stock pot over low heat and whisk well.

2. Continue to whisk over heat until warmed through.

3. Pour into two serving mugs and enjoy!

· SERVING SUGGESTION ·

SERVE WITH COCONUT WHIPPED CREAM AND AN EXTRA SPRINKLE OF TURMERIC IF DESIRED.

Nutritional Information:
Carbs: 8g
Fiber: 3g
Net Carbs: 5g
Protein: 3g
Fat: 36g
Calories: 338

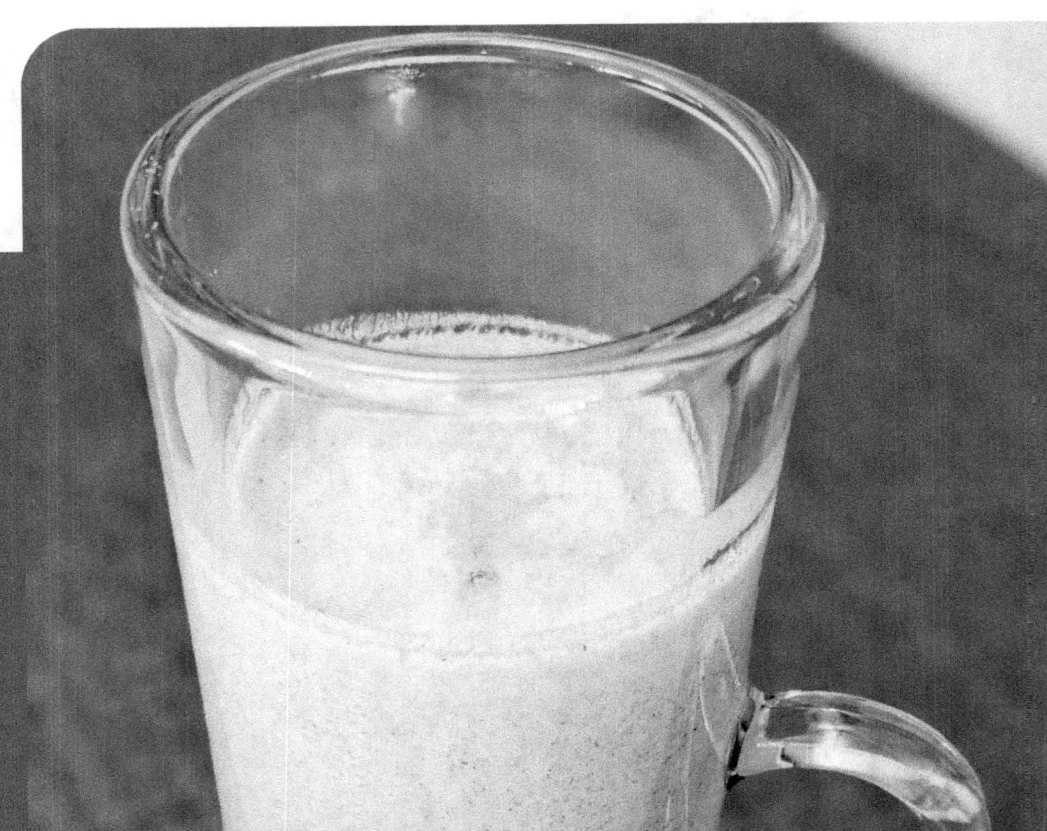

Iced Turmeric Ginger Tonic

Prep Time: 5 minutes
Cook Time: 0 minutes
Serves: 2
Difficulty Level: 1
Cost: $

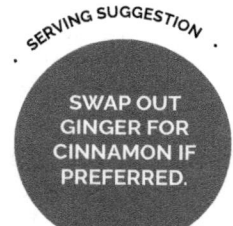

SERVING SUGGESTION

SWAP OUT GINGER FOR CINNAMON IF PREFERRED.

Ingredients:

- 1 cup brewed black tea, chilled
- ½ tsp ground turmeric
- ¼ tsp ground ginger
- 3 drops of vanilla liquid stevia

(or whatever one serving is depending on your liquid stevia)
- Ice

Directions:

1. Add all ingredients to a beverage shaker minus the ice and shake well.

2. Pour over ice.

3. Enjoy!

Nutritional Information:

Carbs: 1g

Fiber: 0g

Net Carbs: 1g

Protein: 0g

Fat: 0g

Calories: 4

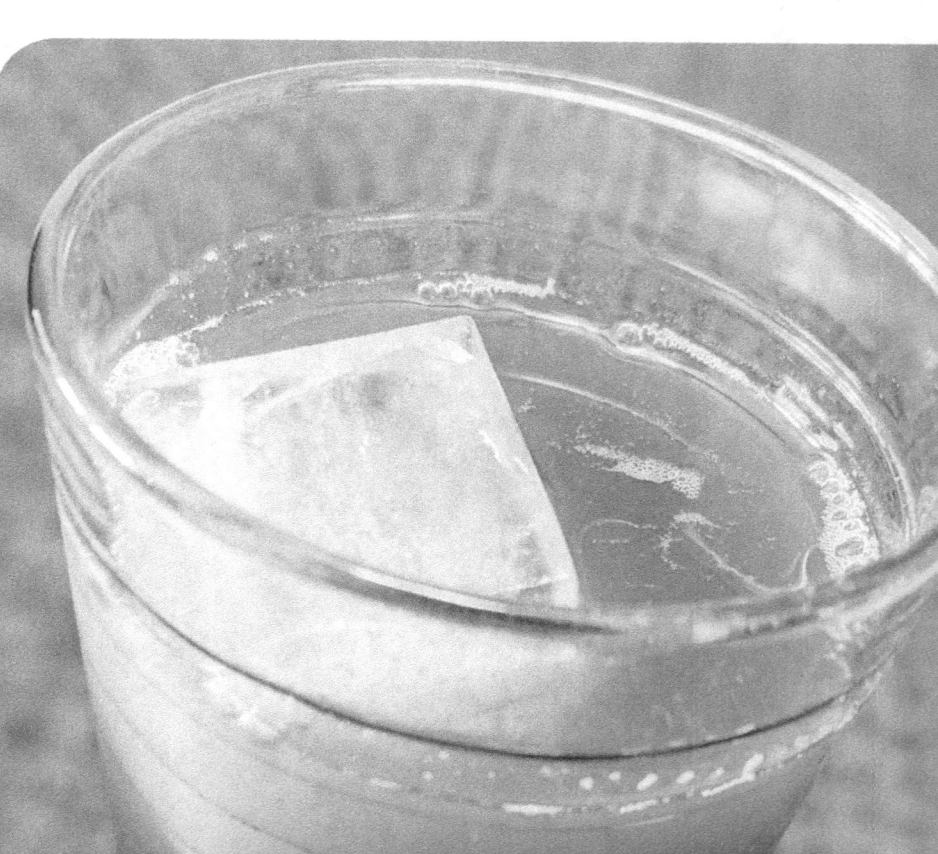

Comforting Chai Tea

Prep Time: 5 minutes
Cook Time: 5 minutes
Serves: 2
Difficulty Level: 1
Cost: $

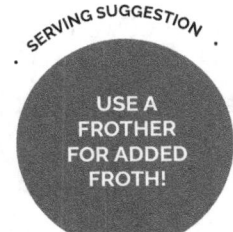

SERVING SUGGESTION

USE A FROTHER FOR ADDED FROTH!

Ingredients:

- 2 chai tea bags
- 12 ounces hot water
- ½ cup full-fat unsweetened coconut milk
- 3 drops of vanilla liquid stevia (or whatever one serving is depending on your liquid stevia)

Directions:

1. Add the chai tea bags to a large mug with the hot water. Steep for 5 minutes.

2. Add the coconut milk and stevia to the mug and whisk well.

3. Enjoy!

Nutritional Information:
Carbs: 1g
Fiber: 0g
Net Carbs: 1g
Protein: 0g
Fat: 3g
Calories: 25

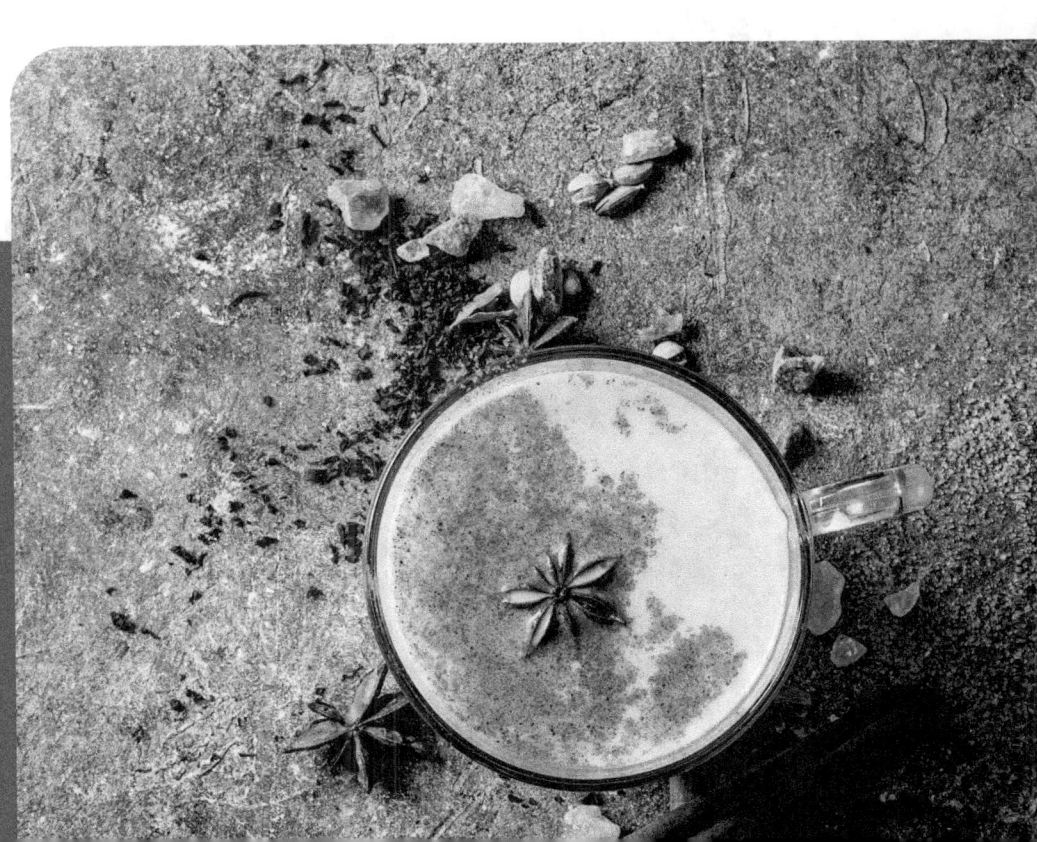

Creamy Coconut Chai Latte

Prep Time: 5 minutes
Cook Time: 5 minutes
Serves: 2
Difficulty Level: 1
Cost: $

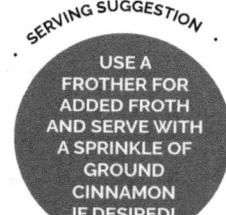

SERVING SUGGESTION

USE A FROTHER FOR ADDED FROTH AND SERVE WITH A SPRINKLE OF GROUND CINNAMON IF DESIRED!

Ingredients:

- 1 chai tea bag
- 8 ounces hot water
- 1 shot of espresso
- ½ cup full-fat unsweetened coconut milk
- 3 drops of vanilla liquid stevia (or whatever one serving is depending on your liquid stevia)

Directions:

1. Add the chai tea bags to a large mug with the hot water. Steep for 5 minutes.

2. Add the espresso, coconut milk and stevia to the mug and whisk well.

3. Enjoy!

Nutritional Information:

Carbs: 4g

Fiber: 1g

Net Carbs: 3g

Protein: 1g

Fat: 14g

Calories: 141

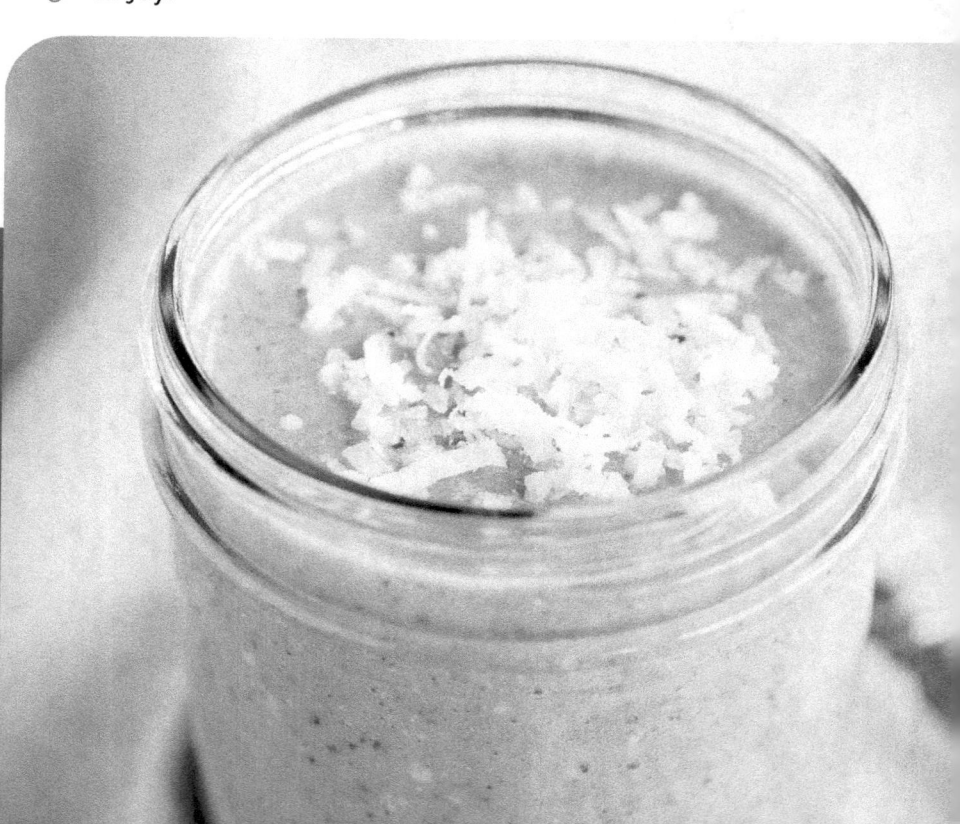

Cleansing Celery Juice

Prep Time: 5 minutes
Cook Time: 0 minutes
Serves: 3
Difficulty Level: 1
Cost: $

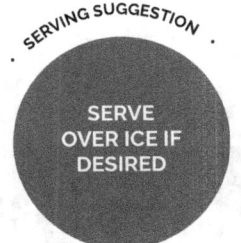

SERVING SUGGESTION

SERVE OVER ICE IF DESIRED

Ingredients:

- 1 bunch of celery
- 1 bunch of cilantro
- 1 lemon, sliced

Directions:

1. Run all ingredients through your juicer according to the manufacturer directions.
2. Serve in a glass and enjoy right away!

Nutritional Information:
Carbs: 10g
Fiber: 5g
Net Carbs: 5g
Protein: 2g
Fat: 1g
Calories: 50

Pomegranate & Lime Spritzer

Prep Time: 5 minutes
Cook Time: 0 minutes
Serves: 2
Difficulty Level: 1
Cost: $

Ingredients:

- 1 tbsp freshly squeezed lime juice
- 1 tbsp pomegranate juice
- 1 cup plain sparkling water
- 3 drops liquid stevia
- Ice

Directions:

1. Start by adding the lime and pomegranate juice to two serving glasses.
2. Add the sparkling water, stevia, and ice.
3. Enjoy!

· SERVING SUGGESTION ·

SWAP OUT THE LIME FOR LEMON JUICE IF DESIRED.

Nutritional Information:
Carbs: 10g
Fiber: 0g
Net Carbs: 10g
Protein: 0g
Fat: 0g
Calories: 39

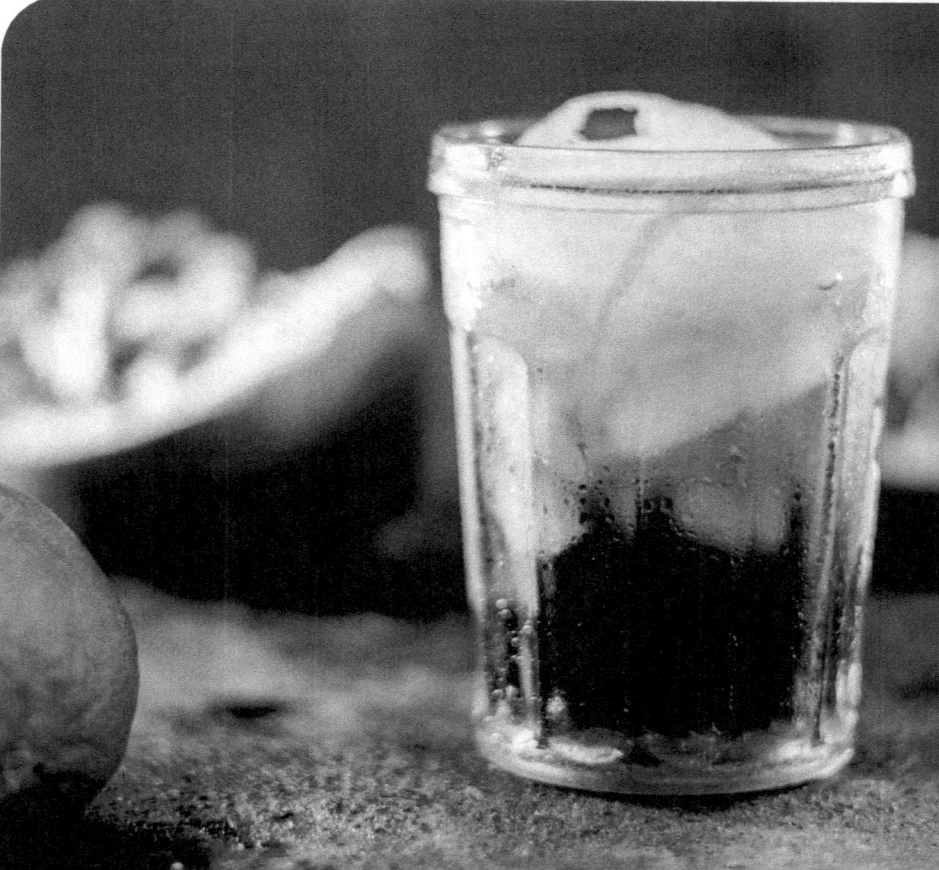

Holiday Peppermint Mocha

Prep Time: 5 minutes
Cook Time: 5 minutes
Serves: 2
Difficulty Level: 1
Cost: $$

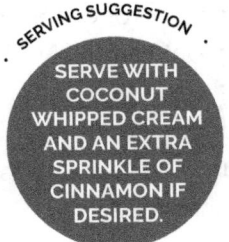

SERVING SUGGESTION

SERVE WITH COCONUT WHIPPED CREAM AND AN EXTRA SPRINKLE OF CINNAMON IF DESIRED.

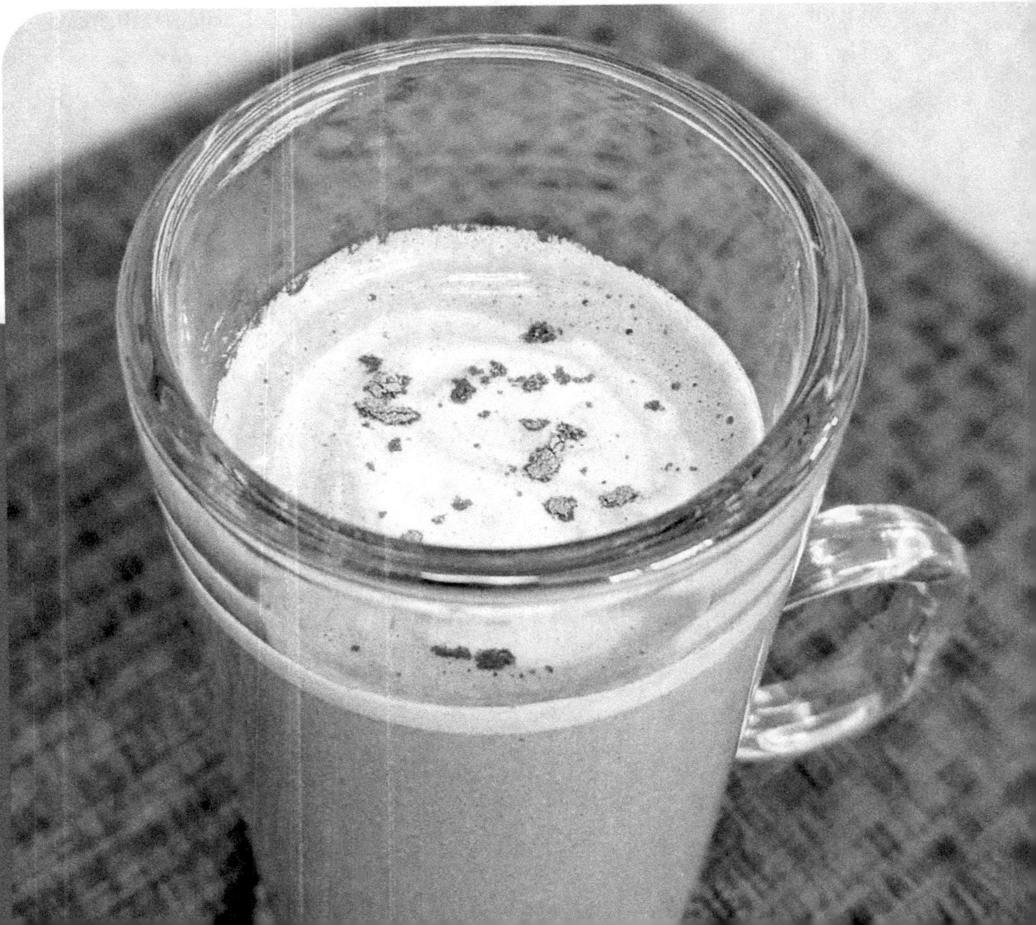

Nutritional Information:
Carbs: 18g
Fiber: 9g
Net Carbs: 9g
Protein: 7g
Fat: 33g
Calories: 329

Ingredients:

- 1 cup full-fat unsweetened coconut milk
- 2 tbsp unsweetened cacao powder
- ½ tsp pure peppermint extract
- 1 tsp ground cinnamon
- 3 drops liquid stevia

Directions:

1. Add all ingredients to a stock pot over low heat and whisk until warm.
2. Pour into two serving mugs and enjoy!

Ebook ISBN: 978-1-953607-27-0
Paperback ISBN: 978-1-953607-28-7
Hardcover ISBN: 978-1-953607-29-4